Why settle for less-gasm?

MORE

G A S M

Babeland's Guide to
MIND-BLOWING SEX

Claire Cavanah and Rachel Venning

Text by
JESSICA VITKUS

Photographs by
SARAH SMALL

Designed by
HEADCASE DESIGN

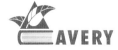
AVERY

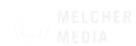
MELCHER
MEDIA

This book is dedicated to

OUR AMAZING STAFF OF BABELANDERS,

OUR CUSTOMERS,

and

ALL THE ORGASMS THAT HAVE COME ALONG THE WAY.

Avery Books
Published by Penguin Group (USA) Inc.
375 Hudson St, New York, New York 10014, U.S.A.

Penguin Group (Canada), 90 Eglinton Avenue east, Suite 700, Toronto, Ontario M4P 2Y3, Canada (a division of Pearson Penguin Canada Inc); Penguin Books Ltd, 80 Strand, London WC2R ORL, England; Penguin Ireland, 25 St Stephen's Green, Dublin 2, Ireland (a division of Penguin Books Ltd); Penguin Group (Australia), 250 Camberwell Road, Camberwell, Victoria 3124, Australia (a division of Pearson Australia Group Pty Ltd); Penguin Books India Pvt Ltd, 11 Community Centre, Panchsheel Park, New Delhi−110 017, India; Penguin Group (NZ), 67 Apollo Drive, Rosedale, North Shore 0632, New Zealand (a division of Pearson New Zealand Ltd); Penguin Books (South Africa) (Pty) Ltd, 24 Sturdee Avenue, Rosebank, Johannesburg 2196, South Africa

Penguin Books Ltd, Registered Offices:
80 Strand, London WC2R ORL, England

Published by Avery Books, a member of Penguin Group (USA) Inc.

Avery Books and the 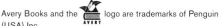 logo are trademarks of Penguin (USA) Inc.

First Printing, January 2010
10 9 8 7 6 5 4 3

ISBN 978-1-58333-372-3
Printed in Hong Kong

Copyright © 2010 Babeland LLC
Photographs © Sarah Small
Text by Jessica Vitkus
Design by Headcase Design

This book was produced by **MELCHER MEDIA**

{ Contents }

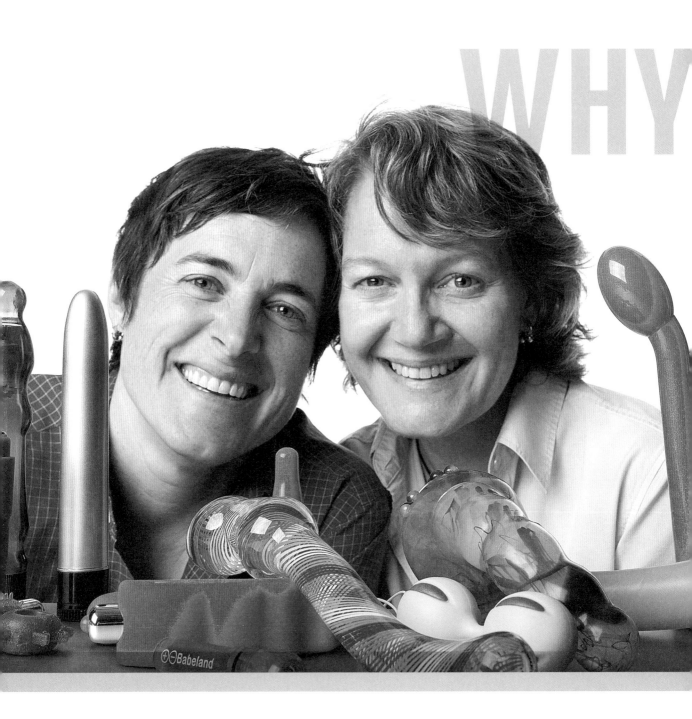

WHY

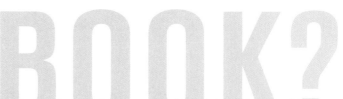

THIS BOOK?

Since 1993, people have been coming into Babeland and asking us questions. "What's your newest toy?" "How do I get my partner to do x?" "Where's the G-spot?" "How can I have a better orgasm?" Or even "I like x, y, or z (being tied up, or fantasizing about being overpowered, or getting toes sucked). Is that normal?"

Babeland is a smart, friendly sex shop where we help people find answers to their questions about sex and encourage their explorations, because who cares what's normal if it feels good?

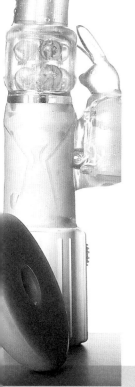

Some of the queries are sophisticated, others are basic. Once, a man came in and asked Claire, "So ... is the clitoris on the inside or the outside?" We're glad he asked, and we bet his future lovers are too! We all have gaps of knowledge and secret curiosities about sex. Whatever you're curious about, keep asking. Because no matter how experienced you are, there are always questions about getting turned on, getting it on, and getting off.

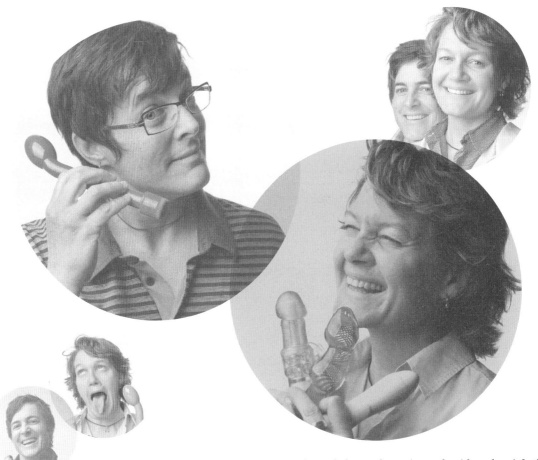

We think sexual pleasure is a joy and a right. At Babeland, the two of us, along with hundreds of Babelanders (our term of endearment for the folks who work here) past and present, have worked very hard to provide accurate, honest info to guide folks—and now you—on the journey to Ecstasy-ville. Everyone's desire is different, and no one figures out great sex automatically. It takes practice, practice, practice. Fortunately, that's practice you can enjoy!

After years of talking with customers, studying up, trying our toys, and running workshops, we've learned a lot about sex. We love passing on the good word. It's fun to help people get in touch with and satisfy their desires. We hope this book helps you get answers and encouragement—sexuality is an important part of life, and the difference between a happy sex life and a bad one is significant. So go for a good one—follow your desires, try new things, express yourself, and explore. This book can be a companion for your journey.

Moregasm tackles the questions we hear all the time, questions we know you're thinking, and others you might never have imagined. You can read this start to finish or just skip to what's on your mind. Dig in!

THIS BOOK'S FOR YOU

It's fine if you like sex with men, women, someone who's a little of both, a vibrator, a dildo, your right hand, a bowling ball, or a mongoose. (Well, there are bestiality laws and health concerns with that last one, but you get the idea.) The sad truth is that in our culture, **female sexual pleasure is underrated and underappreciated.** Just think of any mainstream movie you've seen lately with a sex scene … does the woman have time to get aroused? Lubricated? Does the guy check in to see if she's coming? Does she speak up and tell him, "A little more to the left"? Is there time for her to come again? And do guys ever have a hard time getting an erection? And how about all those ads for penis enlargement and breast augmentation? You see our point. With all these messages telling us sex should be quick, easy, and automatically satisfying, and that our bodies aren't good enough, no wonder people are disappointed by the real thing or settle for less.

So we wrote this book to champion great, realistic sex.

We didn't assume too much—we know you may be doing it with men or with women, and definitely with yourself. We cover a lot about sex with a partner, but a good sexual relationship with yourself is the foundation of super sex with others.

This book is written from a woman's perspective, but it will also help anyone who has sex with women to become a better lover. This is the book we would have liked to have had when we were coming into our own, trying new things, exploring new people, and learning to love sex.

CHAPTER 1

LAY OF THE LAND:

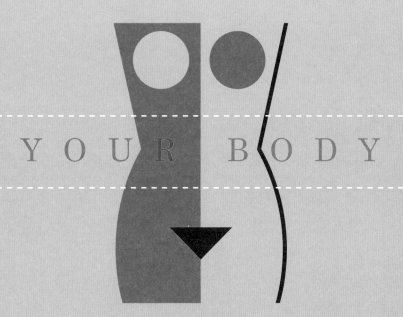

YOUR BODY

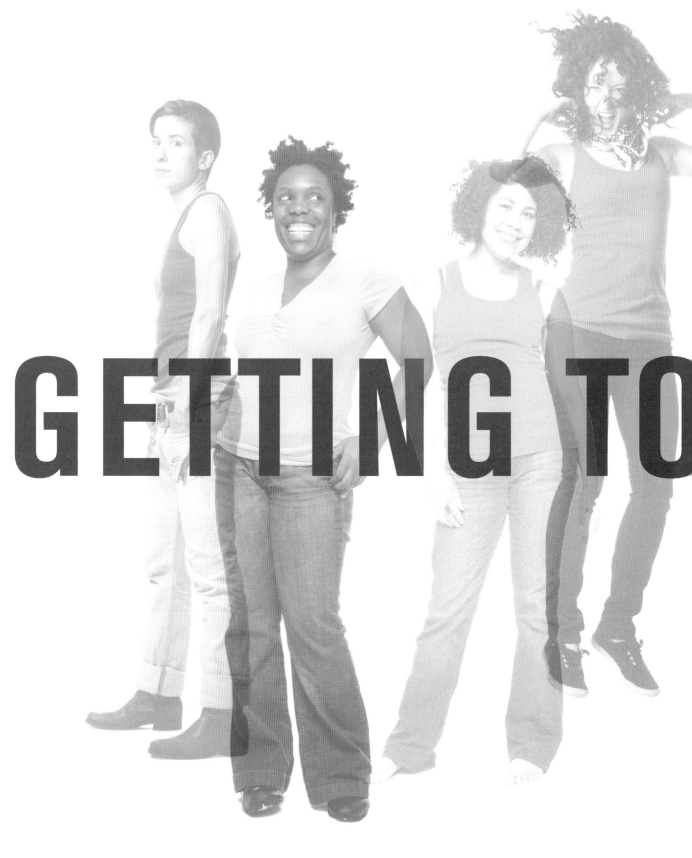

GETTING TO

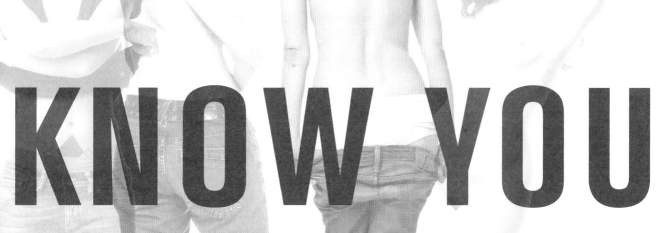

KNOW YOU

Step one on the journey to good sex is learning how your own body works—what it wants, what feels good, what changes occur when you get turned on. How can you tell your partner what to do if you don't know?

Get ready to do some exploring.

(More on masturbation on p. 52.) But before you set out, here are some maps for the journey.

All Your
SEXY PARTS

Good sex doesn't just happen in crotch country. It's a full-body experience, like dancing or sports. The more you use your whole body and coordinate your actions, the more satisfying the performance. All of your sexy parts can get involved—as tools, as objects of beauty, as receivers of touch. And if you have a great orgasm, it rocks you from your scalp to your toenails.

1. LIPS

A crucial tool for feeling your way in the dark, lips are loaded with nerve endings beneath very thin skin. They also engorge when aroused, that is, get fuller and redder (hence the use of lipstick to mimic the look of arousal). You use thirty-four different muscles when you kiss.

2. NECK

Another very sensitive, often neglected area. Are you extra ticklish here? Is your partner? Be sure to explore with fingertips and mouth.

3. BREASTS

The windows to the soul. Just kidding. Lots of folks love sensation on their breasts and nipples—though tastes vary as to what kind: some like hard, some like gentle, some prefer none. It's a very individual thing, so don't count on any surefire "moves" with breast play. The nipple has erectile tissue that firms up when aroused.

4. BELLY

Sure, six-pack abs are hot to some, but so are a lot of other belly shapes. Sex is no fun if you are suck-ing in your belly the whole time. And loving your body is perhaps the sexiest thing you can do; try it and see!

5. BUTT

Many say we are hardwired to get turned on by ass shape. The butt is home to the anus. Though many say "ew," many others say "ahhhh." The A-hole might not have the popularity of the vagina or mouth, but it has nerve endings galore. Some practice, a bit of lube, and a gentle touch can bring fireworks of pleasure. Aren't you at least curious?

6. LEGS

Legs play a powerful part in courtship and attraction. Think of all the body language in how you sit and stand when you fancy someone. Visually, legs are the "highway to heaven," enticing the viewer to think about where they lead. Anyone who's ever put on a miniskirt knows this.

7. KNEES

Behind the knees lives very soft, sensitive skin. Don't forget to enjoy it.

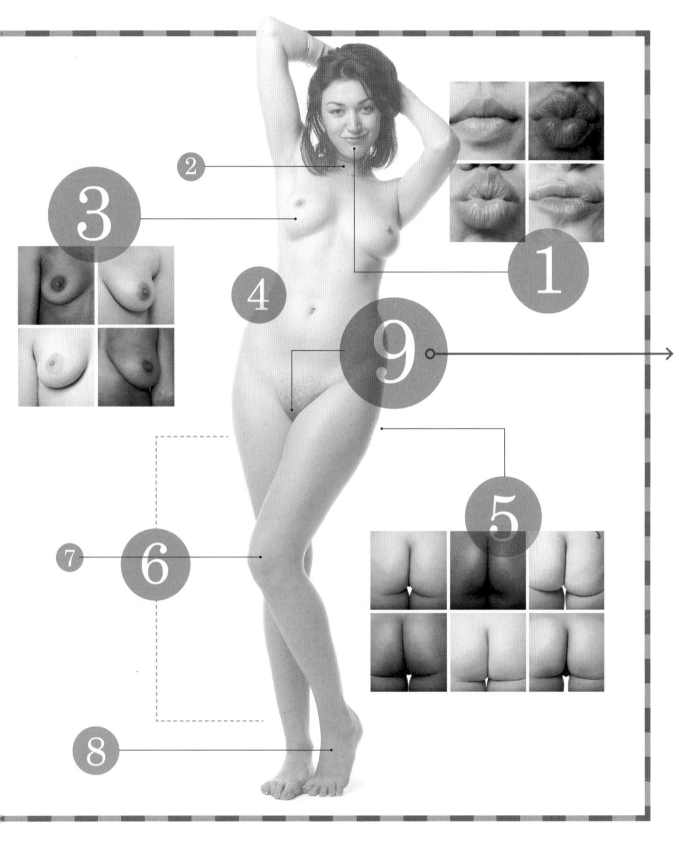

THE SPICE OF LIFE:

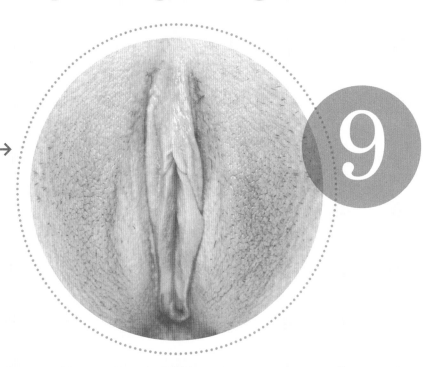

9

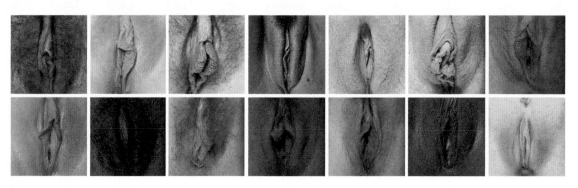

Vulvas come in a range of proportions and shapes and personalities. There's the demure innie and the "hello, sailor" outie. They're not always symmetrical. Check out our gallery of gal parts.

8. FEET

We've locked up these sensitive souls (and soles!) in shoes. Fortunately, the abundant nerve endings are still there waiting for some touch. Just ask a reflexologist … or anyone who's received some sexy toe sucking. There are legions of foot admirers. Some experts think that foot-o-philes get off on the humility of loving the part that touches the ground—kind of like kissing the hem of a queen's robe.

9. VULVA

Vulva means the entire female genital area, the equivalent of "the package" on a guy. Sometimes we just call it the V. Of course, the vagina nestles within the vulva, but it's important to remember all the sensitive tissue and parts around the vagina. Especially the clit! (See p. 18.)

TONGUE (not shown)

While most body parts do just one or two things well, the tongue does triple duty—it can feel, taste, and moisten. It's made up of interlacing muscles that allow you to shorten it, lengthen it, or swirl it all around. Nature's best sex toy.

FINGERS (not shown)

Primates use touch more than any other creature. Our fingertips are packed with nerve endings that are super sensitive to pressure, texture, temperature, and vibration. This made it easier to find the ripest, softest fruit back when we were monkeys. Now those fingertips can feel all the subtle textures and reactions of the body you're touching (whether it's your own or someone else's). In the dark, your fingers become your eyes. And think of all the shapes they can make as givers of touch, and the ways they can move, alone or together.

EARS (not shown)

So sensitive that some paraplegics and quadriplegics can achieve orgasms from oral sex to the ear. And don't forget all the ways that sounds can stimulate—moans, sighs, dirty talk. Arousal causes voices, especially women's, to get lower. Ears love taking that in.

THE VULVA

Everything's Connected in V-Town

Just as all your major body parts work together to make a delicious sexual experience, your vulva is made up of lots of smaller parts that work together when you are turned on. When one little mini-organ wakes up, there's a chain reaction. Soon they all join in the fun and get flush and full and warm with blood. The more you know about the big V, inside and out, the more effectively you can play and enjoy. You may have discovered some of your favorite hot buttons by happy accident, but here's a guide to help you find even more.

EXTERNAL { Figs. A, B }:

1. VULVA

A name for all of the visible external parts: the mons pubis, the labia, the clitoris and its hood, and the vaginal and urethral openings.

2. MONS PUBIS

Loosely translates as "pubic hill." This is not a bushy city park. It's the mound of flesh right over the pubic bone where hair grows. Underneath the mons pubis lies the ligament that holds the clit in place, so massaging this area or grinding the pelvis against something (a hand, a pillow, a good friend) can be pleasurable.

3. CLITORIS

A.k.a. "the man in the boat" or "the love button." The clitoris is much like a mini-penis. It has a head and a shaft and gets erect when excited. And it's bigger than it looks, as it has legs that extend several inches under the labia toward the vag.

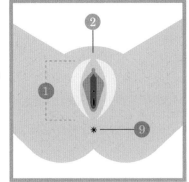

{ Fig. A } EXTERNAL VIEW

The head can vary in size and shape and in how much it shows. This visible nubbin has more than 6,000 nerve endings. The clit is the only human body part designed purely for pleasure. Most women need clitoral stimulation—direct or indirect—in order to orgasm.

4. CLITORAL HOOD

A small sleeve of protective tissue that covers the clit—the equivalent of a foreskin on an uncircumcised penis. Some hoods cover a lot, and the clit hardly shows. Other hoods are barely there, and the clit says "hello." Some women like clit stimulation through the hood because direct touch is just too intense.

5. OUTER LABIA

These are the outer lips that cushion and protect the tender parts beneath. They are mostly fatty tissue with some hair. The outer labia are less sensitive than other parts of the V.

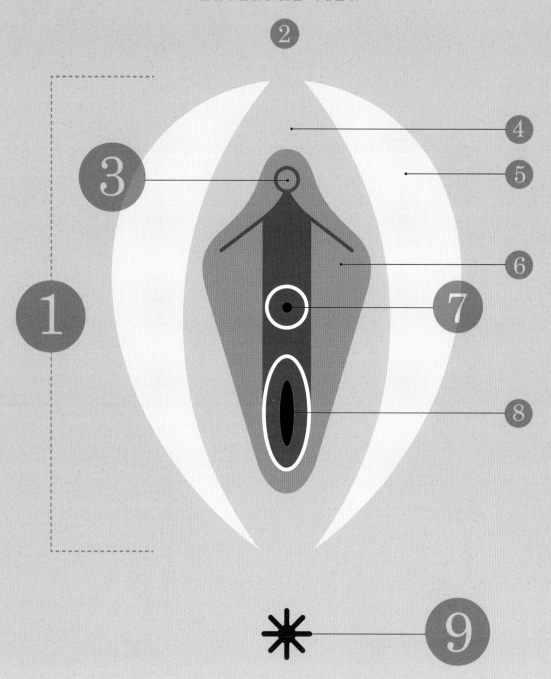

{ Fig. B }
EXTERNAL VIEW

6. INNER LABIA

Inner labia are hair-free and much more nerve-rich than the outer labia. They swell when excited and attach to the head of the clitoris—so stroking them can stimulate the clit. Inner labia can be small and tucked in or big and blossoming out. They can appear dark or light in color.

7. URETHRA OPENING

The entrance to the urethra.

8. VAGINAL OPENING

The entrance to the vagina.

9. ANUS

There is lots of fun to be had here. See p. 26 for more information.

INTERNAL { Fig. C }:

10. URETHRA

The thin tube that carries urine away from the bladder and out the urethral opening. The urethral opening can be small and hard to find. Since bacteria can migrate here during sex, be sure to pee afterward—nature's flushing system.

11. URETHRAL SPONGE

Spongy erectile tissue that wraps around the urethra, protecting it. It contains lots of glands. During arousal, blood flows into the spongy tissue, and the glands fill with fluid. This is most likely the fluid that squirts or puddles out during female ejaculation.

12. G-SPOT

Here's where you can feel the urethral sponge through the vaginal wall. It's tough to find when a woman isn't aroused, but when she is, the urethral sponge gets big and full, and there's a place about two inches into the vagina on the belly side that feels like a rough, spongy walnut. Bingo. Some love having their G-spot stroked or massaged with fingers or a vibrator. Others find it annoying.

13. VAGINA

The passageway to (and from) the uterus, made of two muscular walls that rest against each other. It helps to think of the vagina as more of an envelope than a tube. At rest, it's only about four to five inches deep. During arousal, the walls of the vagina get flush with extra blood and become moist for smoother entry of fingers/penis/toys. The first couple of inches of the vagina contain most of the nerves. Excitement makes the rear part of the vagina swell, lifting it another two inches or so. The deeper part is less sensitive but responds to pressure and "fullness."

14. HYMEN

A thin, often crescent-shaped membrane just inside the vaginal opening that stretches across like Saran Wrap—with a gap along the top so you're not sealed off like a yogurt container. After puberty, the hymen gets thicker and more elastic, with a bigger gap. Tampons and fingers can get in and out more easily. Contrary to myth, the hymen doesn't necessarily go "pop" and bleed with your first sexcapade. It can tear from tampons or fingers or reasons we don't know. It often happens in stages and not in one big painful swoop. Leftover bits of hymen can remain as loose tags. If you experience pain during intercourse because of these remnants, see a doctor.

15. CERVIX

A knob of firmer tissue in the back of the vagina that serves as the gateway to the uterus. In the center, there's an opening—called the os—where menstrual blood flows out or sperm can go in. The cervix gets softer and more sperm-friendly during ovulation. It

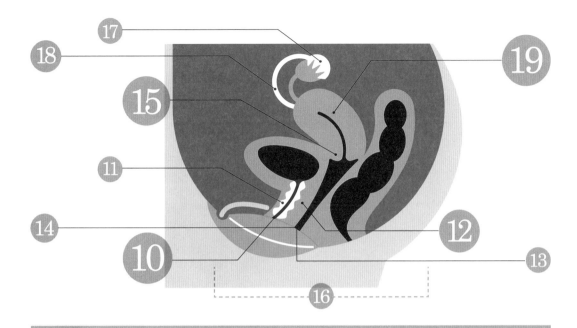

{ Fig. C } INTERNAL VIEW *The objects in the mirror are closer than they may appear! To give you a better sense of your insides, the above illustration shows more space between the urethra, vagina, and anus than actually exists. In reality, the urethral sponge is right against the vagina's wall, and the wall between the rectum and the vagina is also very thin.*

also releases mucus that can help block sperm or welcome sperm into the os—depending on the time of the month. If a thrusting penis or dildo bonks the cervix during sex, it can hurt or it can feel great—depending on how you're wired.

16. PC MUSCLE
Short for pubococcygeus, it's a muscle system that forms the bottom of the pelvic floor, holding up the bladder and the uterus. During excitement, the PC muscle contracts involuntarily, and it outright spasms during orgasm. You can also control and play with your PC muscle for greater pleasure. (See Kegels, p. 23.)

17. OVARY
About the size of an olive, there's an ovary on each side of the pelvis. Ovaries produce eggs. The two ovaries take turns releasing a mature egg (or "ovum") each month. Ovaries are analogous to the testes in men.

18. FALLOPIAN TUBES
Like the tunnel from Brooklyn to Manhattan, fallopian tubes provide a pathway for the egg from the ovary to the uterus.

19. UTERUS
Shaped like an upside-down pear, the uterus has three entrances—a fallopian tube on each side (where eggs come in), and the cervix (where sperm come in). This is where the egg ends its journey each month. If the egg is fertilized, it nestles into the lining of the uterus and develops into a fetus. The uterus (a.k.a womb) stretches like a balloon during pregnancy. If the egg is not fertilized, the lining sheds—a.k.a your period.

MIRROR, MIRROR, ON THE FLOOR ... WHERE'S THE VULVA I ADORE?

Compared with dangly man-parts, female genitalia is more internal and out of sight. Why not take a closer look at yours? Yes, it kind of smacks of 1970s feminist consciousness-raising groups, but where would we be without those? Just put on your love beads, grab a mirror, and either squat over it (which leaves both hands free) or lie back and spread 'em (holding the mirror in one hand). Make sure you're in good light. Match yourself up to the V-map (p. 19). Try this solo or invite your partner to explore with you.

WHAT DO A CLITORIS AND A WISHBONE HAVE IN COMMON?

Answer: their shape.

YOUR CLIT HAS LEGS

The head or the glans of the clit is what peeps out, then there's a shaft about the thickness of a drinking straw. You can feel it if you wiggle your finger just above the hood—an inch or two of ropiness from the glans up toward your belly button. Good news: the fun doesn't end there. The clit splits into two legs (called crura) that run down each side of the vaginal opening. Shallow penetration and fiddling with the inner labia can make the clitoral legs happy. They swell up like the rest of the clit when excited. And the whole thing is shaped like a wishbone.

KEGEL-ROBICS

The PC muscle is the one you clench to stop the flow of pee. You can exercise this muscle group and reap a lifetime of benefits. Namely, stronger, better orgasms. The PC muscle is what holds all the tension that builds up during the thrust and grind of sex. The stronger the PC muscle, the more tension it can hold, and then the greater the explosion upon release. Hooray! You'll also increase blood flow and sensitivity. An added bonus: you'll have a sturdier pelvic floor during pregnancy and reduce your chances of incontinence later in life.

These exercises are called Kegels, after the doctor who made them famous. If you start clenching your PC muscle, you'll notice that you can tighten around the vagina and around the butt hole. You can clench both areas together or separately. Lean forward a little and clench to flex your vagina, and lean back a little to feel the anal part. Try these exercises anytime—in line at the post office, at Thanksgiving dinner, or during your boss's sales presentation. No one will know.

1 The Catch-and-Release

Inhale and clench at the same time. Hold both your breath and your clench for a few seconds, then release both.

2 The Flutter

Contract and release your PC muscle ten times in a row. Rest a few seconds and repeat.

3 The Plumber

Inhale and contract both your vaginal and anal PC muscles as if you were pulling in water. Hold, and on your next inhale, contract more, as if you were pulling the water in deeper and higher. Do this for four or five breaths, then release and push your PC muscle as if you were shooting out water. For fun, try doing it with just the vaginal or the anal part of the PC muscle. How does it feel?

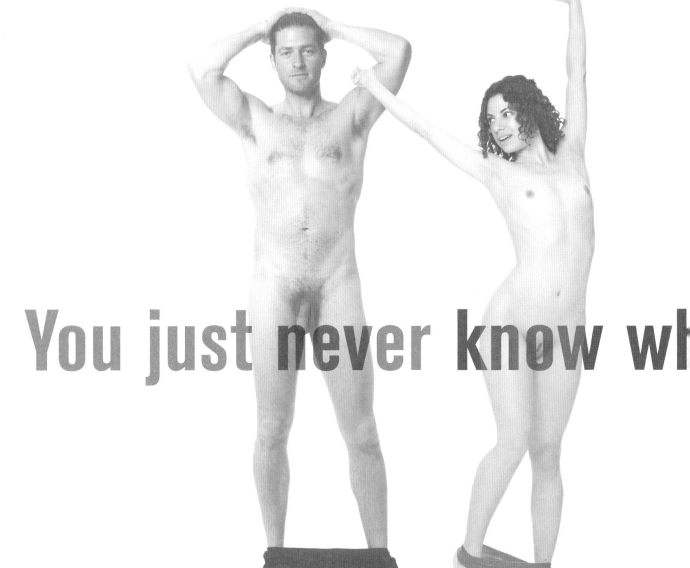

You just never know wh

LIKE BROTHER, LIKE SISTER

Male and female sex organs may look totally different, but in the womb they all start out the same. Until
about eight weeks, all embryos have the same little
protogenitals. If male hormones kick in, boy genitals
develop. If not, the embryo remains a girl. Once you
know this, it's easier to understand the analogous
parts in men and women. For example, the same
nub of fetal tissue develops into either a penis or a
clitoris—both organs have a head and a shaft and get
erect when excited. The same fetal tissue grows to be
either foreskin on the penis or a clitoral hood. The
scrotum is like the outer labia. The prostate gland is
analogous to the urethral sponge. Interesting, no?

TRANS & GENDERQUEER & INTERSEX

Some bodies don't fall neatly into the "male" or "female" categories. One or two out of two thousand babies are born with elements of both boy and girl genitals. Intersex people have aspects of both male and female characteristics. Not a surprise, considering male and female sexual organs are sculpted from the same fetal materials. Each of us is assigned a sex at birth. In fact, it's usually the first thing that happens when we enter the world. Doctors and midwives proclaim with utter certainty, "It's a girl!" or "It's a boy!" when they see a baby's genitals. And most of us grow up feeling more or less aligned with that first

t's in someone's pants

take on our gender. But some people don't end up feeling like their genitals and their identity match, and they might choose to change their bodies with hormones and/or surgery to feel more completely at home. For example, someone born female might have a bilateral mastectomy and take male hormones that cause the clit to enlarge. This person might look, dress, and identify as a guy, but he still has a vulva, although he may choose to rename it to match his male identity more closely. So the two-party system of "male" and "female" doesn't quite work. There's a range of possibilities in between. And you just never know what's in someone's pants until you're lucky enough to be invited in!

YOUR BUTT

The Friendly Next-Door Neighbor

Your anus is right next door to your vagina, so it would be downright rude to ignore it. Why not at least introduce yourself? Blood flow, nerves, and the PC muscle all connect the V-hole to the A-hole. So why not bring it a little love? Understanding the parts will help you understand how to make it feel good.

EXTERNAL { Fig. A }:

1. CHEEKS

The muscular padding we sit on. The cheeks appreciate a different kind of touch than the genitals or anus. Kneading and massaging are nice. This helps get the blood flowing and the muscles relaxing near the tender parts. A good spank on the lower region of the cheeks can also resonate nicely all through the genitals.

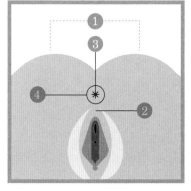

{ Fig. A } EXTERNAL VIEW

2. PERINEUM

The stretch of skin between the vagina and the anus in women or the balls and the anus in men. Sensitive. Often ignored or underrated as a place to tickle or massage or touch with a vibrator.

3. ANUS

The opening that leads to the rectum and then the colon. The area around it is loaded with nerves and sensory receptors—so licking and massaging and sending vibration there all feel great. When the anus is relaxed and excited, blood flows to the area, and it even puckers out a bit.

4. OUTER SPHINCTER MUSCLE

This muscular ring is mostly under your control. It lets you decide when and where to take that poop (thank you, outer sphincter!). It needs lube and loving in order to open the gate.

INTERNAL { Fig. B }:

5. INTERNAL SPHINCTER MUSCLE

A muscular ring that can open and close like the drawstring on your laundry bag. Located about an inch inside the anus, it lets you know when poop has arrived and is ready to be "dropped off at the pool." The inner sphincter is not a voluntary muscle. It does its work automatically. In fact, it responds to unwanted poking by tightening up and even hurting. This ring needs to be

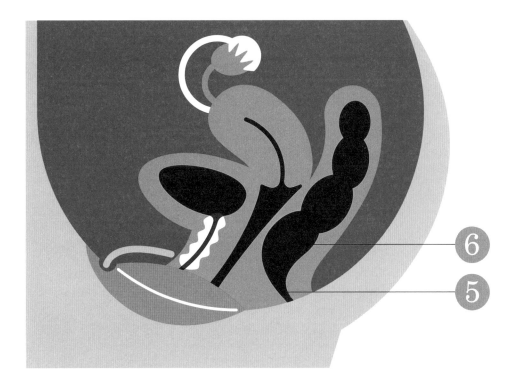

{ Fig. B } INTERNAL VIEW *Remember, your rectum is not a cul-de-sac, as our diagram might lead you to believe. That means no marbles up the butt!*

really relaxed and happy and lubed in order to let a finger/toy/penis through. There's simply no rushing or forcing it.

6. RECTUM

The chamber just inside the outer sphincters. It goes about eight inches in a shallow S-curve up to the colon. The wall between the rectum and the vagina is thin enough that you can feel through it. Many people like the feeling of fullness when the rectal walls are holding something like a finger, butt plug, dildo, or penis. Normally, the rectum is empty. Poop lives farther up in the colon until it's time for release. Yes, there can be traces of poop in the rectum, but nothing you can't wash off with a little soap and water. Try a warm water anal douche if you want to be extra clean. If you choose to clean out your rectum, you can use a saline enema from the drugstore, but usually a shower beforehand is sufficient.

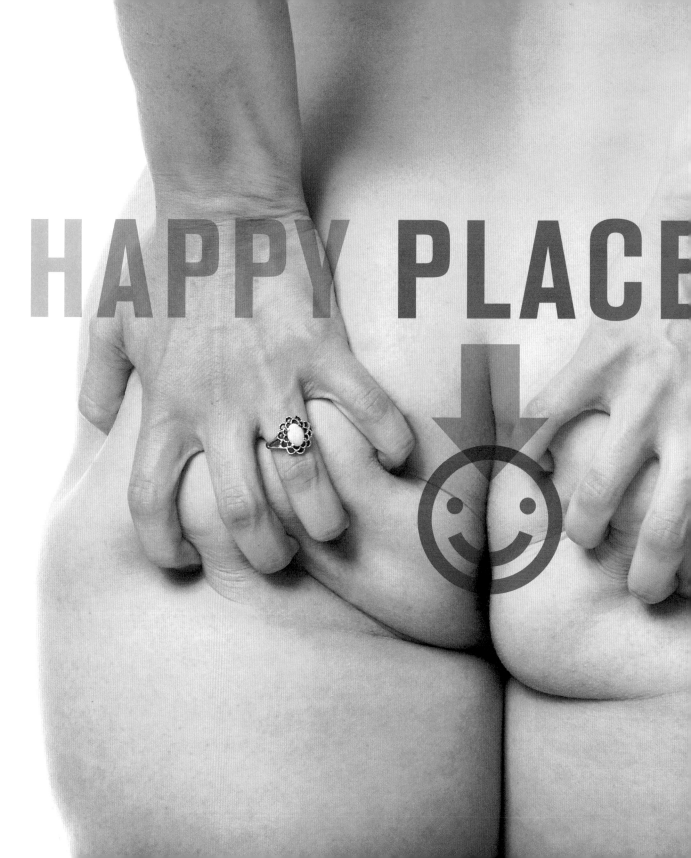

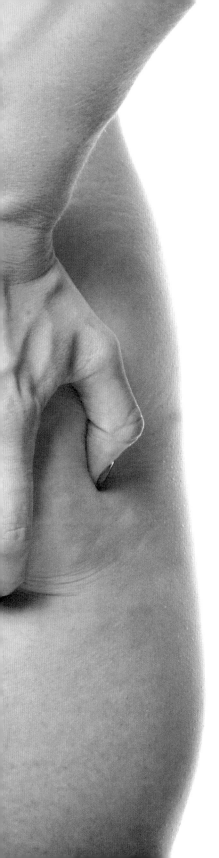

IT'S GOOD FOR YOU

In our culture, we hold a great deal of tension in our ass muscles, including our sphincters. The term "tight ass" was coined for a reason. So anal play (which doesn't have to mean penetration—a little lubed massage is a treat in itself) can help you release this tension and unwind. Think how good a shoulder rub feels after a tough day. Why not soothe your butt hole too? And, contrary to popular belief, anal sex does not cause lasting incontinence. In fact, the opposite is true. Gentle stimulation and exercise of the sphincters will more likely help keep these in/out valves working longer, letting you walk on by the Depends aisle.

SOME NOTABLE DIFFERENCES

The anus is a great place to play. But you can't treat it like the vagina. Anatomically speaking, we urge you to keep these differences in mind during sex play:

• NO LUBE, NO LOVE

The anus does not create its own lubrication. Adding extra lube is a must. Saliva won't do it. You don't have enough, and spit dries up quickly.

• THIN-SKINNED

The tissues of the anus and the rectum are thinner and more fragile than those in the vagina. Even the slightest hangnail can make a significant scratch, and scratches in there are more likely to bleed. It's easier to transmit an STI through the anus, too.

• NOT A DEAD END

We are all for putting toys up your bum. But the anus doesn't have a back wall for safety like the vagina does—it goes on and on, up into the rectum, which leads to the colon. Don't lose your insertables. Only use toys with flared ends or strings for easy removal. (More on anal-sex play in Chapter 6.)

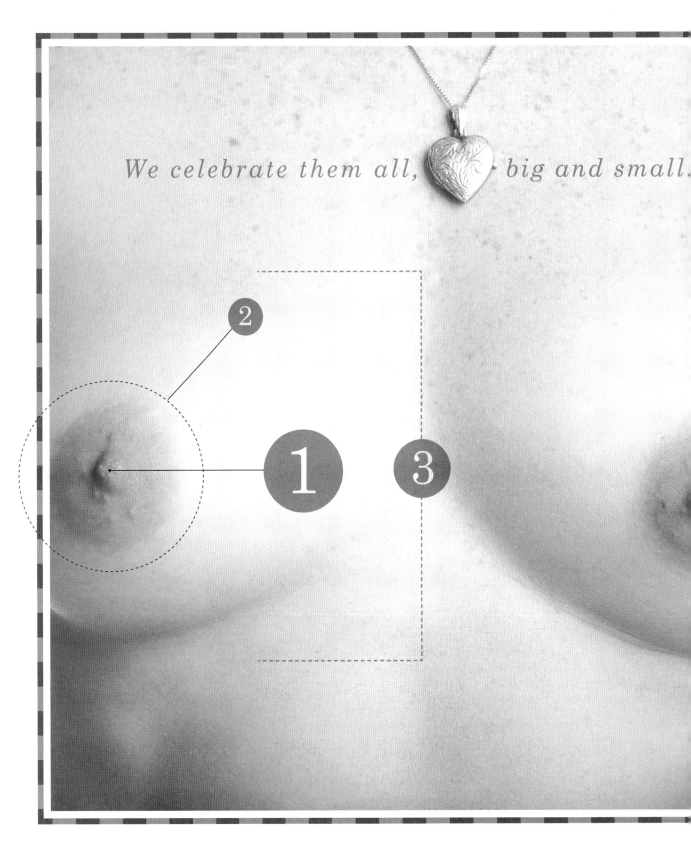

We celebrate them all, ~ big and small.

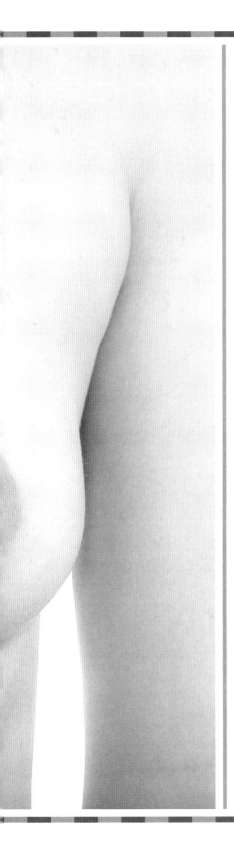

[YOUR BOOBS]

The Girls

Dress designers, film directors, and straight teenage boys have all worshipped at the altar of the boob. Breasts can represent comfort. They can entice and turn on. Here's how they work.

- -

1. NIPPLE

Loaded with nerve endings, the nipple is a sensitive button. It's where all the milk ducts lead. Some lucky women feel like their nipples can bring fireworks of arousal. Others find nipple play annoying.

2. AREOLA

The darkish circle around the nipple. The areola can be brown or pink or tan or barely there. It can be big like a saucer or small like a coin. It can stick out a little like an acorn top or lie flat. It might have hairs growing around the edge (you can pluck 'em or leave 'em). All normal. The areola is sensitive to touch and kissing and sucking.

3. FATTY TISSUE

Much of the breast is simply fat. (That's why boobs sometimes get smaller if you lose weight.) The fat content starts low in young breasts, then increases with age.

MILK GLANDS AND DUCTS *(not shown)*

Mammary glands are made up of milk-producing areas and ducts. These ducts carry the milk to the nipple when a woman is nursing. If your breast feels lumpy and ropey, you are probably feeling the milk glands and ducts (though the fat can be lumpy, too). Get familiar with your own breast texture so you'll notice any changes later in life.

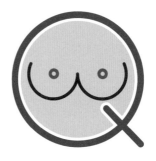

{ Q & A }

BOOBIE QS

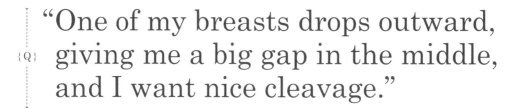

{Q} *"One of my breasts drops outward, giving me a big gap in the middle, and I want nice cleavage."*

{A} After one day of reading magazines and watching TV, almost any woman might want to turn in her own mammers for a new set. Round, high, and immune to gravity is not the way nature made most of us. Look around at boobs when you are shopping at the grocery store or out with friends. Enjoy the variety. Not only is there a range of breast shapes and sizes but their placement on the body varies from one woman to the next. (See p. 15.) The way breasts sit on the rib cage will affect how they fall. Your rib cage is probably more convex, so the breasts fall outward. A good push-up bra can create cleavage where there is none, but a low-cut V-neck that just shows acres of skin between the boobs is sexy too. It's worth coming to love what you have. You are a babe, and your chest is part of your total babeliness, whatever it looks like.

"A light touch on my boobs is just not enough."

{Q}

{A}

Some women are turned on by just a soft breath on the nipple. Others don't feel much until you basically use a clamp from a woodshop. Your boyfriend or girlfriend may be doing things that made some other breasts very happy. But the lessons they learned on other women aren't always transferable. The good and bad news is that every new set of girls means starting over and discovering what makes them feel good. It's a fun challenge, and you can help. Since your lover probably isn't the Breast Whisperer (who is?), give some guidance, maybe demonstrate with your own hands, and give lots of positivity when you feel something you like.

"I want breast implants. Should I get them?"

{Q}

{A}

First off, we bet some women with big breasts would envy you. You don't have their back pain, and you can wear lots of clothes that the be-hootered can't. Breast implant surgery carries risks, and after the surgery the implants can burst or migrate or cause scar tissue. You can also end up with reduced breast sensitivity, which seems like a big sacrifice. Can you make peace with the pair you've got? Think about the positive feedback you have gotten from partners (we bet they were more excited to caress your breasts than to measure them). There are all kinds of delicious padded bras and bra inserts that might make you feel sexy. But if you are convinced that only implants can make you feel happy and vital and alive, then go for it.

"Why are my breasts extra sensitive at some times and not at others?"

{Q}

{A}

Breast sensitivity varies from day to day. Menstrual cycles can affect the boobs—they can get super sensitive to touch around ovulation or right before your period. Birth control pills can also cause sensitivity. In all these cases, breasts are responding to a change in hormone levels. This can mean your breasts are loving life, or it might mean "keep off!" Try tracking your cycle in your date book to figure out the pattern. The more you know about yourself and your body, the better. It's empowering! It will also be easier to clue in your partner so they aren't baffled by any game change.

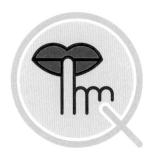

{ Q & A }

AESTHETICS
and
INSECURITIES

{Q} "My inner labia hang out.
I heard there's labiaplasty
I can get for this."

{A} Inner labia that show are totally normal. The artist Georgia O'Keeffe painted flowers inspired by the beauty of labia. Unless they're causing physical problems or pain, please don't clip your little wings. There are rare cases where longer labia can get caught and pinched during sex—and that's no fun. Labia are sensitive and deserve tender care, not a scalpel unless absolutely necessary. Yes, there are a few doctors who do this procedure. There are also doctors willing to give you a "G-shot"—that's a hypodermic needle to inject collagen into the G-spot. These doctors make us want to break windows. Say no to unnecessary elective procedures on your V.

34 |

"Why do I have a pubic bush, and what should I do with it?"

{Q}

{A} The short answer is: just do what makes you feel sexy. The longer answer is: pubic hair probably evolved as a place to capture our musky smells, as those smells are important to finding a mate and making a chemical connection. You (or your partner) might like the visual of an untamed bush growing free. Then there are degrees of trimmed hedges. You can keep your shrubbery in check with small scissors (like mustache scissors), or you can use electric beard and mustache trimmers that have a V-friendly plastic protector on the end for safety. (Shout out to the Wahl Clipper Corporation, which makes one of our best-selling plug-in vibrators!) Some folks like the look of a bare vulva—you can see the outer labia—and there's a sexy feeling of exposure to it. And someone going downtown on a bare V doesn't get pubes in the teeth. Or you can wax or shave yourself a landing strip, or a heart, or your lover's monogram. Have fun! Just be aware that both waxing and shaving can cause bumps and irritation. Get waxed by a total pro, and do your shaving with utmost care, moving the razor in the direction the hair grows, not against it. There are also products to soothe skin and prevent bumps. If you are feeling sassy and brave, let your partner shave you.

"I'm worried about my scent. What should I do?"

{Q}

{A} Your pussy smell and your skin smell are all part of the chemical magic that is really a form of communication. Have you ever taken a sniff of a T-shirt a partner wore and left at your house and found it exciting? Your genitals have a smell that can be sweet, acidic, musky, or some combination. We bet you'll meet someone along the way who loves it. Your "eau de vagine" can change a little with diet, your menstrual cycle, and even stress. Get familiar with your own smell—you've done the old touch-'n-sniff on yourself, right?—so that you'll notice when something is awry. A new and bad smell can be a sign of infection, namely bacterial vaginosis, or BV. BV is easy to diagnose and treat, but you should either see your doctor or treat it with natural remedies. Otherwise it could become something worse. Bottom line, we bet your pussy smells...like a pussy. Keep it clean by rinsing in the shower. Use mild soap. If it makes you feel better, you can use perfume- and soap-free wipes before someone gets up close and personal.

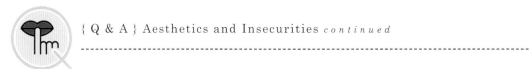

{Q} "I'm a little insecure about getting undressed in fron

{A} We all feel self-conscious sometimes, and of course taking your clothes off makes you feel vulnerable. Why do you think we have dreams (nightmares) of being naked at City Hall or a class reunion? The good news is that your new partner is probably so excited to get busy with you, they are probably not focusing on that ill-timed butt zit. Or even better, they might find your little imperfections charming. Would a butt zit wreck the game for you? We bet not. Here are some tips—both practical and spiritual—for feeling good naked.

• GROOM AND LET GO

In other words, control what you can and let go of what you can't. Clip your nails, trim your bush, exfoliate, etc., and then don't worry about your crooked feet or your appendectomy scar. (P.S. Scars are sexy. They tell a story.)

• VISUALIZE THE HAPPY EVENT

That's what athletes do before the big game. Combine this with meditation and slow breathing if you like. Picture the two of you touching each other and digging it. Let it play out in your head like a delightful movie. It's a little like rehearsal and makes for a nice fantasy—that can come true!

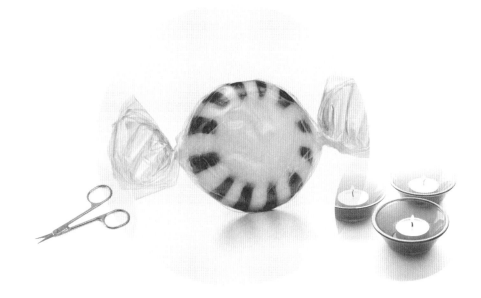

my body and I dread of a new lover. Ideas?"

• CHOOSE GOOD LIGHTING

Ask any filmmaker or restaurateur: lighting can make anything look sexier. We love candles. Especially ones that melt into massage oil.

• BE CANDY

When the time comes to disrobe, pretend that you are unwrapping a delicious piece of fine candy.

• FOCUS ON YOUR BODY SENSATIONS

Get out of your critical head and notice the sensations of your body—is your cunt juicier, is your skin tingly, does the air smell good?

• FOCUS ON THE OTHER PERSON

If you focus on making the other person feel sexy and turned on, you'll forget your own worries. This is a good time for your rock-star oral sex technique, maybe.

• THINK ABOUT TRUST

If you don't feel like this person is going to accept your nakedness with happy open arms, then maybe it's too soon. Maybe it's not the right person.

CARE AND FEEDING *of your* LADY PARTS

Your vagina has a built-in cleaning system. The vaginal mucus you find in your panties every day has a pH balance that helps fight germs and bacteria. It's your first defense against infection. So you don't want to mess with that internal system. Keep all the surfaces clean and healthy, and avoid trapped moisture, which can irritate this tender region. Some Babeland dos and don'ts:

- **DO** use mild soap, or no soap, when washing your V. Don't use body gels or overly perfumey soaps. A lot of folks just use water!

- **DO** clean your V with your hand (or a volunteer's hand!), not a washcloth, which can trap bacteria. Be sure to clean between the labia and under your clitoral hood. Gently. Pat (don't rub) dry.

- **DO** wear cotton underwear, because it breathes.

- **DO** wipe yourself front to back after pee or poop. This keeps butt germs away from the urethra and vagina.

- **DO** sleep naked. Nighttime is a great time to let air circulate.

- **DON'T** wear pantiliners on your non-period days. They trap moisture and keep it pressed against you.

- **DON'T** use harsh laundry detergent or lots of laundry detergent. Traces of it in your undies can irritate your V.

- **DON'T** wear nylon or acrylic tights. They trap moisture. Thigh-highs are healthier and way sexier.

- **DON'T** even think about douching or using feminine spray, perfume, or baby powder on your V.

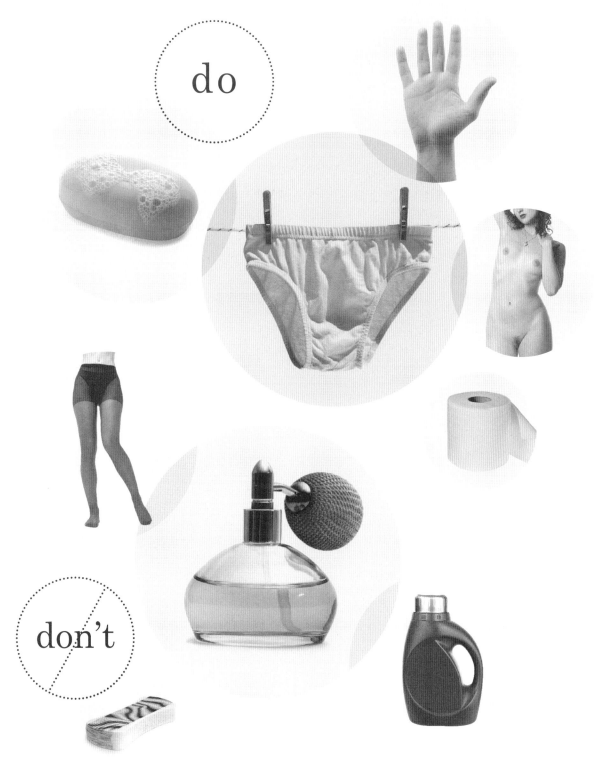

do

don't

CHAPTER 2

LOVE THYSELF:

THE BIG O,

MASTURBATION, *and* TOYS

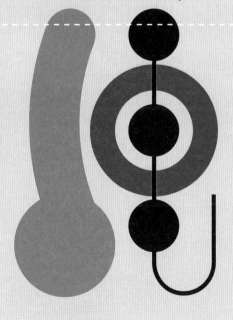

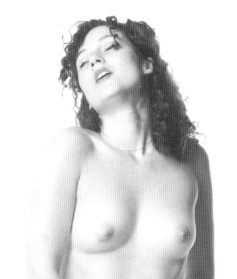

BE THE MASTER OF

Now that you've gotten to know your body a little better, it's time to start exploring how to find your **sexual pleasure,** which we think **is every woman's birthright.** Orgasms can be elusive, for sure. At **Babeland,** we don't think it's enough to just cross your fingers, pray to the gods, and **hope one comes along.** It's not fair to leave the job 100 percent to your partner (though they are clearly welcome to help!). We nominate all of you to **be in charge of your own orgasms.** Actively. As with most

YOUR UNIVERSE

worthwhile things in life, **you've got to work a bit in order to reap the rewards.** You will get out of it what you put into it. Sometimes a minimal-effort quickie is just what you need. Other times a date night with yourself is better. And if you've had a rough week and really need a Happy Ending (the naughty kind), we want you to have it. Whether you orgasm at the drop of a feather or just once in a while—or even if you haven't had one yet—**we can help you**...to help yourself.

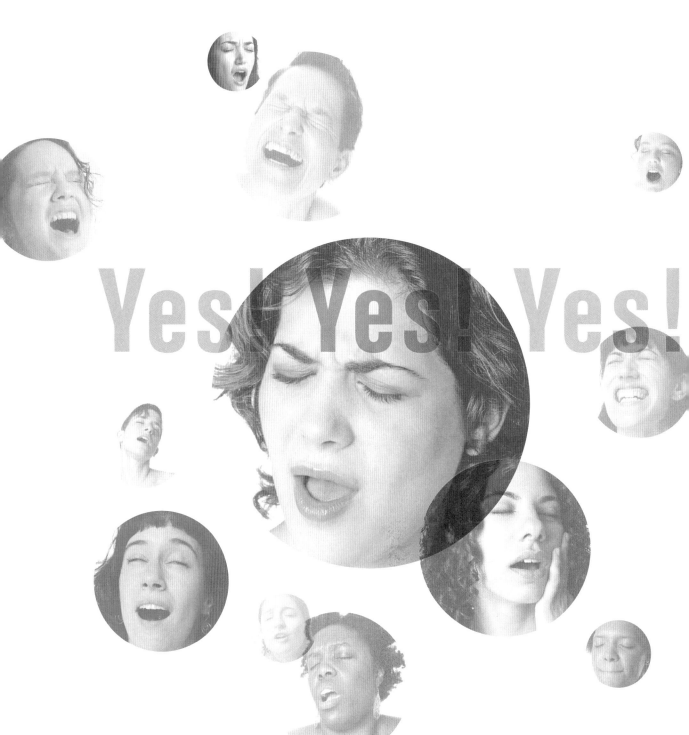

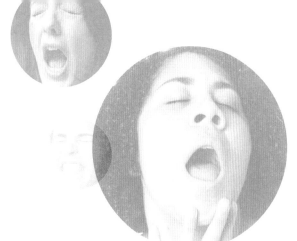
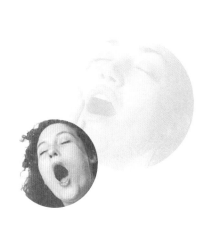

Oh, Yesssss!!!!!

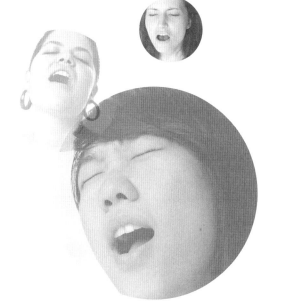

O IS FOR ORGASMS

Orgasms are wildly different for everyone—especially women. Coming can feel like an inside-out earthquake, a swooping roller coaster, a warm light all over, or a million other metaphors. (Note: we are fairly certain that an orgasm does not feel like a shampoo commercial.) Orgasms can be brief, like a jolt, or long and flowy. For some women, there's even ejaculation! Orgasms can also be small and quiet. And within one person's sex life, Os can come in degrees and varieties. They are the opposite of boring.

YOUR ORGASM

We'd be crazy to spell out the "typical" or "normal" orgasm. We don't consider any sexual response normal or abnormal—we think of sex as more of a garden full of variation and beauty. What's a normal orgasm? What's a normal flower? There are some common physical changes that you can be on alert for, though you may not feel every one of them. Whether you're alone or with a partner, tune in and try to notice what sets you off, what ups the ante, and what makes you lose yourself. Is it a certain fantasy? A certain rhythmic touch? A certain visual image? A special hot spot?

CLIMBING THE HILL

The stages of an orgasm are not separate like stair steps. Each blurs into the next—more like climbing a hill. You won't always make it to the top, and you may not always want to. Be patient with yourself and honor what you want every time you're getting it on.

Stage One: Arousal

As you begin to feel aroused, your heart beats faster, which causes increased blood flow to the nipples and vulva and breasts and lips. You might feel warmth all over and flushed skin. Muscle tension increases. Your vagina starts to get wetter, while the clit and labia swell up a bit. The vaginal walls respond to the excitement by making more room inside, the space ballooning back as the cervix lifts. You probably feel more sensitive to stimulation all over and significantly less sensitive to pain. Check out, for example, what your nipples are up to. Are they saying, "Oh my God, a tickle feels like an electric shock"? Or are they saying, "Grab on, honey, and let's go for a ride!"?

Stage Two: Plateau

The feelings from the arousal stage continue and intensify: blood rushes to the vulva, which gets excited and engorged, along with the clit, labia, and urethral sponge. You feel a tightness and sensitivity and overall tension. Your clit retracts under the clitoral hood. You might begin to feel a sense of climbing, floating, or flying. Deeper breathing at this stage can create erotic energy and spread the feeling of arousal from the groin to the entire body.

Stage Three: Climax

Your heart rate and breathing intensify. You feel a series of involuntary muscular contractions in the vagina, uterus, pelvic floor, and beyond. You might also feel contractions in your butt muscles, your arms, and your face—almost anywhere, since it's all connected. Your whole body may shudder. You may ejaculate fluid. There are usually three to fifteen contractions (whose job was it to count?). These muscle spasms release blood from the engorged tissue, returning it to the rest of the body and resolving the feeling of tension. The brain releases a cocktail of neurochemicals that make you feel anywhere between good and transformed.

Stage Four: Resolution

Your heart rate, breathing, and blood pressure return to normal. The flushing of the skin (often on the face and chest) disappears. The vulva returns to its previous size. If you were excited but didn't climax, it will take longer for you to return to your regular state. Many women are blessed with the ability to continue on to more orgasms from this state. In guys, ejaculation typically includes the loss of the erection, so they're done until the cycle starts again. In addition to other neurochemicals, a dose of oxytocin (a.k.a. the Cuddle Chemical) kicks in. That's the one that bonds a breast-feeding mother and child. With resolution can come feelings of relaxation, sometimes the release of tears (with or without sadness), looseness in the joints, and a feeling of being right with the world.

P.S. At this point, after you come, that same delicious clitoral touch that helped bring you or your lover to orgasm might feel very irritating. Ouch! Time to focus on something else. There are times when the clit will go to the overstimulated place even before the climax stage. The clit just needs a rest—you can come back to it later.

. . . AND DON'T FORGET DESIRE

Doctors and sex therapists used to start this flow chart with another stage: desire. Desire has its own physical responses, like dilated pupils. But the problem is, you can experience desire and not feel ready for sex. You can have the symptoms of arousal but not feel any desire (like the teenage boy who gets an erection during math class). It's also possible to begin having sex while being a little bored and not that into it, then feelings of desire kick in later. So that's why desire was booted off the chart. Perhaps it's further proof that our minds and bodies can get really out of sync.

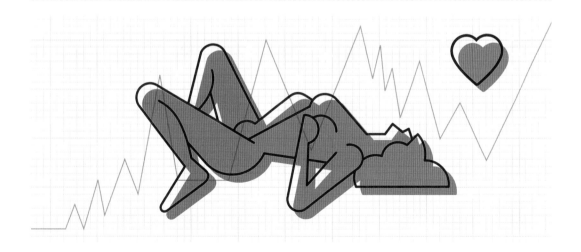

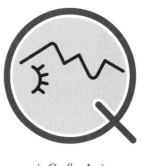

O REALLY:
THE ORGASM QUESTIONS

{Q} "What's the difference between a clitoral and a vaginal orgasm?"

{A} Two thirds of women do not orgasm from vaginal penetration alone. In other words, most women need direct clit stimulation to rock their world. Freud said that clitoral orgasms were "immature" and vaginal orgasms were "mature." But we respectfully call that a load of B.S. Modern scientists generally agree that, technically speaking, an orgasm is an orgasm—how it resonates in the body is not based on where the stimulation came from. In fact, orgasms from vaginal penetration do involve the clit, because the legs of the clitoris reach back and around the vaginal opening. So… clitoral or vaginal? They all sound like good orgasms to us.

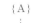

"My orgasms don't look like the ones in porn."

{Q}

{A}

Forget porn. How about just regular R-rated movies? Or reruns of *Sex and the City*? The media sets up unrealistic expectations. An orgasm is something happening internally. But these performers have to communicate their pleasure externally. The actors want the people in the cheap seats to get the message "I'm coming!" so they moan and squawk and writhe and flail. And they somehow manage to remain attractive through it all. Please don't let that be a model for how you (or your partner) should look or sound when you come. In fact, not worrying how you look or sound will help you orgasm. Yes, you make faces and funny sounds. Or you might be quiet and spazzy—what does it matter? If making noise helps you get there, go ahead and wake the neighbors! Part of the joy of partner sex is letting yourself be vulnerable with someone else. Part of the joy of masturbation is letting go any way you want.

"What does pre-orgasmic mean? Is that me?"

{Q}

{A}

We think nearly all healthy women are capable of orgasm in one form or another. Being pre-orgasmic means you have not had an orgasm yet or are not sure if you have. Since there are so many ways a climax can feel, we understand if you're not sure. Especially if you've had sexual encounters (solo or partnered) that felt really, really, really good. The key question is: have you felt the involuntary muscle spasms? If not, or if it happens only once in a while when the stars align, we think you can change up the game. You've got the equipment. You might want to find new ways to play. Try a powerful plug-in electric vibrator for the best chance of success. And give yourself more practice time. (See Masturbation, p. 52.)

"Is it possible to orgasm without genital stimulation?"

{Q}

{A}

We're big believers in whole-body sexuality. Sexual response isn't located in just our genitals. Bring in more parts of your body, and you'll feel enlivened and can even have whole-body orgasms. If your clit or vulva is not responsive, you can still get off with stimulation to other parts of your body. People with different abilities, including people with spinal injuries, certain diseases, or other issues, can enjoy a sexuality as robust as anyone's, including orgasm without genital involvement. Even if your clit is fully functional, it's great to expand your areas of exploration.

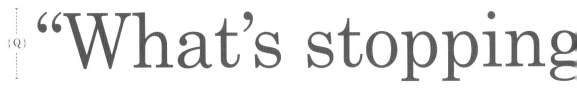

{Q} "What's stopping

{A} This is a big question, so the answer won't reveal itself overnight. But take a moment for a little self-diagnosis. These are some common obstacles people face. If you pinpoint what's bugging you, you can start to focus on it and face it. Which of these might be getting in your way?

• KNOWLEDGE GAP

If you are not coming, learn about your body and know what to touch. If you are only trying penetration, you'll have better luck if you focus on the clit. Building arousal can also take some time—emotional or social pressure (even from just yourself) to come quickly can actually make that sought-after release harder to get.

• BODY IMAGE

It's hard to get out of your head when you are worrying about your body issues. Meanwhile, your partner is probably admiring your ass and dying to feel it. But nonetheless, we are surrounded with unrealistic examples of bodies and unhealthy messages (like "Never too rich or too thin!").

• PARTNER ISSUES

Maybe your partner isn't patient. Maybe your partner doesn't communicate. Maybe your partner isn't the right partner. Find a more communicative, kinder lover, and you'll have way better sex.

• EMOTIONAL ISSUES

If you have suffered sexual abuse, physical abuse, betrayal, or bad sexual experiences in the past, then it can be hard to let go and trust a partner. It can even be hard to let go and enjoy sex by yourself. This one can be too big to manage alone, but there are amazing professionals who can help.

• RELIGIOUS AND CULTURAL HANG-UPS

Did your church or your parents teach you that sex before marriage is a sin? Do you feel guilty having sex for pleasure? Somewhere in your soul, do you feel that enjoying sex makes you a slut or a pervert? These messages are definitely out

me from coming?"

there: think of the girl in every horror movie who gets murdered because she's having hot sex in the woods.

• MEDICAL ISSUES

Many medications affect desire and performance. If you are on medication that keeps you from getting wet, for example, try some lube. If your meds slow down your libido, you can start the act of having sex or masturbating, and sometimes the mojo will catch up or kick in a little later. If not, you can stop. Maybe health problems are getting in the way. Talk to your doctor about your limits and what you can do to move past them or, if that's not possible, to accept them.

• SHYNESS

We don't just mean keeping-the-lights-off shyness. Do you cringe when there's too much attention or focus on you? Like maybe you don't deserve it? Do you worry that you are taking too long, but you dread speaking up or taking action? Shyness can be solo too—you might feel ashamed to focus on yourself. Give yourself permission to feel good. You deserve it. We all do.

• FEAR OF PREGNANCY OR STIs

It's definitely hard to relax and enjoy sex if you are stressing about the outcome—thinking ahead instead of enjoying the moment. This one is easy to fix with birth control and safer sex practices. It's reasonable to expect your partner to take some responsibility here too. Talk about it. If you are having a hard time stopping the action to use birth control and latex barriers, be strong, you're worth it.

• STRESS

This is a major and epidemic O-stopper. The everyday stress of bills and work and life can definitely follow you into the bedroom. Sometimes the end of the day is the most stressful, when you are making mental to-do lists for tomorrow. Try scheduling sex (solo or partnered) for the morning or after dinner if your head is clearer then. Sometimes sex can be like exercise: it seems easier to lounge around watching TV, but once you do it, you think, "Oh my God, that felt good. I gotta do this more!"

MASTUR

THE GREATEST LOVE OF ALL

BATION:

In our store and in this book, when we talk about having sex, solo sex counts. In fact, we consider it **THE BASIS FOR A VIBRANT, SATISFYING SEX LIFE.** You can have a very robust sex life all by yourself. Masturbation is a glorious lifelong pursuit. Because guess what: wherever you go, there you are. Why not empower yourself to feel amazing when you want to feel amazing? Even if you have a partner, is this person with you on every business trip? Or home every time you are in the mood? Impossible. We are all hardwired to feel sexual desire, and if you can light your own fire, you'll be a happier person. Depending on someone else to give us sexual pleasure makes us vulnerable. **SO TAKE MATTERS INTO YOUR OWN HANDS.**

JACKING OFF IS EASY, JILLING OFF CAN BE TRICKY

Women need to learn to get themselves off—and there's no single surefire way to do it. Stimulate the clit? Sure, but directly or indirectly? What kind of motion? Should there be something in the vagina too? What position is good? The task can seem daunting. Some lucky women stumble onto a way to get off at an early age. Maybe climbing a pole at the playground or dry humping during a make-out fest, then suddenly… an accidental or semi-accidental launch into orgasm. (Even then, it takes work to re-create the launch while solo at home.) But most women have to experiment on themselves and find their own way. Create your own solo sex test kitchen and see how much fun experimenting can be!

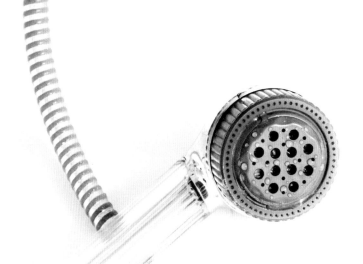

LET ME COUNT THE WAYS

Women masturbate all kinds of ways. As long as you are enjoying yourself and no one is getting hurt, we say go for it. Besides the obvious manual jilling off and the beloved vibrating friend, some other popular ways to polish the pearl are: using water jets (a shower massager or jets in a hot tub aimed at the clit), humping a pillow (lying on your stomach and grinding against the pillow), enjoying the rhythmic movements of horseback riding, sitting on a bouncy clothes dryer, riding a motorcycle, or crossing your legs and squeezing the thighs together (sometimes around something like a pillow). We have one customer who swears she can orgasm from clenching and unclenching her PC muscle while riding a jostle-y subway. We think that's a fine way to commute.

TOP TEN REASONS TO MASTURBATE

1   **DOES A BODY GOOD.** When you are wound up and tense, a good self-induced O relieves the muscles, increases blood flow, and ultimately relaxes you.

2   **EXPLORE FANTASIES.** This is your time to think about any partner you want. Watch any kind of porn that you fancy. You have complete freedom to follow your true desires. Enjoy! See what you learn about yourself.

3   **BETTER PARTNER SEX.** Once you are able to make yourself orgasm, you can teach your partner how to do it.

4   **CHANCE TO TEST-DRIVE.** If there's something you want to try with your partner—a toy, anal play—maybe do it solo first to get an idea of what works and what you like.

5   **RELIEF FROM MENSTRUAL CRAMPS.** 'Nuff said.

6   **SELF-RELIANCE.** No need to badger your partner for sex or spend late nights surfing Craigslist for hookups. If you want it done right, do it yourself.

7   **KEEP THE CHI FLOWING.** Erotic energy is part of our core vitality. Masturbation keeps that energy flowing.

8   **WORLD PEACE.** Dedicate your orgasm to a cause or a person who needs some love. Or just use that O to release some of your own aggression and frustration.

9   **NO MORE PROCRASTINATION.** Is there something you need to get done but you can't seem to get off your ass and do it? Masturbate. It's great for changing gears in your day. (This works best at home, though we have customers who swear they find ways to pet their pussies at work.)

10   **PLEASURE IS ITS OWN REWARD.** Why ask why? A solid sexual relationship with yourself gives you good sexual self-esteem and keeps your whole sexual being running smoothly.

The Basic How-Tos of
MASTURBATION

There's no one way to get off. But if you're having trouble finding your own orgasm, here's a good path to follow. Explore the terrain and find out what feels good to you. Though we are huge fans (the hugest!) of vibrators and toys, we also encourage using your hand for two reasons: 1) Your hand is a two-way communicator that can both feel and give you feedback, and 2) Your hand is always with you—it's nature's sex toy. Have a go.

1. SETTING THE MOOD

Find time when you can be all alone, with no interruptions. Turn off your phone or BlackBerry. Do whatever makes you calm and relaxed, like lighting candles. Make sure the room is a good temperature for getting naked. It's nice to take off all your clothes so you have access to lots of skin. Settle in somewhere you can relax—your bed, your couch, a bathtub full of steamy water. Have some lube nearby.

2. TURNING ON

This step is personal and individual. You can conjure up memories of amazing sexual encounters from the past. You can imagine fantasy encounters with the person you choose (your boss, an actor, the gas meter reader) in the setting you choose (a bordello, an airplane, the White House). You might prefer to read erotica—classics like *Delta of Venus* by Anaïs Nin or *The Story of O*, or new erotica collections like *Best Women's Erotica*. If you have an extra tough time letting go of thoughts swirling in your head, a porn movie can help. Since it gives you visuals and sounds, there's more to pull you in.

(BTW, we sell cool ones made for women.) Porn's not everyone's cup of excitement, but it can be worth a try for fantasy fodder.

3. GETTING STARTED

While still fantasizing or watching your porn movie, find a comfortable position where you can reach yourself. Touch yourself lightly. Tickle your breasts, thighs, behind your knees. You probably wouldn't want a partner to jump right in on your genitals. Same goes for you. Ease into it. Notice which areas are the most sensitive and responsive. Try different kinds of touch: caressing, stroking, kneading, lightly scratching with fingertips.

4. GETTING GOING

When you are definitely turned on, start exploring your V-zone. You may be wet at this point, but a little lube will make for more slippery fun. Some suggestions: stroke your whole vulva in different ways—up and down, in circles, or a figure eight. Vary the speed and pressure of the stroke. Try massaging up and down the inner labia with one or two fingers.

Approach the clit through the hood at first because it's so sensitive. You can stroke up and down the shaft from over the hood. Again, try different speeds and pressure. Notice what feels good and what feels neutral or boring. Feel free to shift positions: legs apart, legs tightly together, feet together and knees apart. Some women prefer kneeling or getting on all fours (really "all threes" if you're using your hand to stroke). Try inserting a finger or two or three into your vagina to see if that feels good. If the clit longs for direct touch, give that a whirl.

5. GOING TO TOWN

Keep changing it up until you hit on a stroke or movement that feels so good you need to keep doing it. Stick with it and find a rhythm. It could be a very small, focused gesture of one finger on the clit, or the heel of your hand vigorously kneading your mons. You can rock your hips to take some of the work away from your hand. Remember to breathe. Make some noises, like moans, which will help you breathe and send feedback and vibration to your body. Most likely, you'll feel the buildup of tension, like you are working or reaching toward something, or like there's a balloon filling up with more and more air before it bursts. This is the plateau stage. Stay here for as long as you like. Stop here if you want.

6. LETTING GO: ORGASM! (OR NOT)

When the tension is built up to the point where you can't take it anymore, just let go. Sometimes you don't have a choice, and your body sweeps you over the edge of the cliff. Sometimes you have to make the decision to give in to your body, to surrender the control. And only then can you come. Orgasm by yourself is a special treat—a time you can be 100 percent unself-conscious. You don't have to think about turning on a partner, or their reaction, or doing anything for anyone. Just let'er rip, baby! Other times, you'll get close but never make it over the precipice. That's totally commonplace. Just remember what felt good.

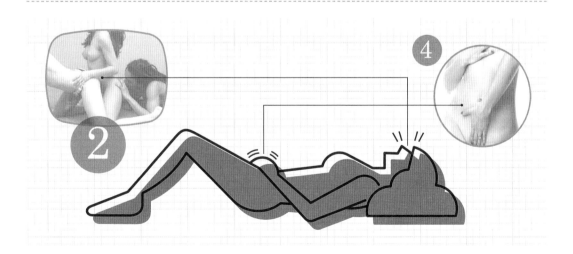

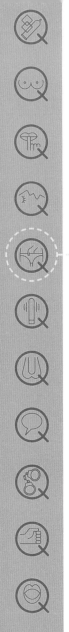

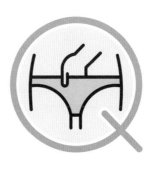

UNKNOWN-ISMS ABOUT ONANISM

{Q} "I always masturbate the same way. Should I mix up my routine?"

{A} Not necessarily. First of all, kudos to you for finding at least one technique that works. If you want to, just go on enjoying your tried-and-true way as long as it's satisfying. We worry that people feel pressure to try wild and wacky things in bed. That's actually not our goal. We want people happy, and we want them to have options. That said ... you might get bored after a while and consider some new moves. You probably have partner sex in all kinds of positions, with different speeds and styles. If you are ready for something new, why not switch it up during solo time?

{Q} "I like to stick a finger up my butt during masturbation. Is that weird?"

{A} No! We're big fans of anal pleasure, and we support your technique. (You're lubing up the extra finger right?) The anus is sensitive and loaded with nerves that are happy to add to your orgasmic pleasure. The anus is so close anyway—it's already enjoying all the extra blood flow and excitement. Maybe even explore more. Many women (and men) enjoy a butt plug during masturbation. Or even a vibrating butt plug (see p. 227).

"I get stuck at the plateau right before climaxing. It's really frustrating."

We hear this a lot at our orgasm workshops. And of course it's frustrating. When this happens, try stopping for a while. Stop masturbation for at least a few minutes and maybe even a few days. Don't dwell on the almost-ness or beat yourself up. When you try again, do this: love yourself up into the plateau state, then back off to a mellower state. Get close to climax and then back off. Repeat as necessary. Then one time, when you get close to the edge, just change things up. Try a new position or a new stroke. Hopefully, this will tip you over the edge. If not, try again another day, or, if you haven't already, experiment with a vibrator (hello, Hitachi Magic Wand!). The strong, consistent stimulation of a vibrator has helped millions of women orgasm. And by the way, the get-close-to-climax-then-back-down-then-repeat exercise is good for anybody. It helps strengthen your PC muscle and makes for bigger, more satisfying Os.

"What's the G-spot, and how do I use it?"

The G-spot is named for Dr. Gräfenburg, an intrepid explorer who published work about it in the 1940s and '50s. Of course, it was there long before Dr. G came along (though many doctors still dispute its existence—feh!).

The G-spot is a cushion of tissue along the vaginal ceiling about two inches in (see p. 20). This cushion is actually the underside of the urethral sponge, which gets engorged with fluid during excitement. Some women love stimulation there. Experiment during masturbation to see if it rocks your boat. When you are already turned on, try inserting two or three fingers. Reach in and try to feel for a patch on the front wall of your vag that's a little rougher and firmer. The G-spot is for stroking, not poking. Stroke it as if you are making the "come here" gesture with your fingers. Experiment with pressure. You might hear angels sing, or you might go "eh." If you hear angels, you can teach your partner to do it. You can also purchase one of the many lovely toys that will help you reach your own G-spot more easily (see p. 74).

"Is there such a thing as female ejaculation?"

Oh, yes indeedy, there is! Sometimes the fluid that fills the urethral sponge ejaculates out the urethra during orgasm. It can squirt water-gun-style or gush like a burst pipe. We swear it's not pee. It's a harmless, clear fluid akin to prostate fluid in a guy. Like sweat, it isn't stored in our bodies but is created quickly when the time is right. You may make a little or a lot. If you want to try to ejaculate, pee beforehand, then get yourself turned on and into the plateau state. Then you (or a partner) should crook the fingers and stroke your G-spot with firm pressure, making a "come hither" motion. Fucking also works for many people, with stiff fingers, a penis, or a dildo rubbing on the G-spot area. At some point, it might feel like you are going to pee. If you feel the urge to pee, don't stop yourself. Let 'er rip. That gushing release may turn out to be part of a stronger orgasm that you've never let yourself have. So if you can take a leap of faith and let loose, you might get a mega-orgasm with waterworks!

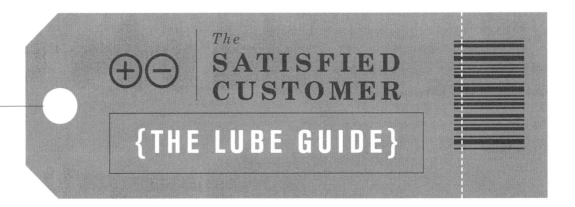

The SATISFIED CUSTOMER

{THE LUBE GUIDE}

There's good friction and there's bad friction. And lube always causes good friction. Sometimes your own juices are not flowing enough—which may or may not reflect your level of excitement. It's good to have lube nearby in case you need it. It's like salt at a meal—keep it handy in case you need a little something extra. It makes your sex play more slippery and fun, and it's a great complement for toys and safer-sex supplies. Don't just take it from us. Here's what some loyal users have to say.

"I WANT A SCENT-LESS LUBE."

Try BabeLube, which has only four ingredients. This gentle lube is tasteless, odorless, and latex-compatible.

What our customers say:

"BabeLube is beyond great. I had been using a popular lube that did the job but was drippy, sticky, and as it turns out, causing a lot of irritation because of the glycerin. I didn't think it was possible, but this lube just dries to nothing. I actually think this lube improved my marriage."

"I WANT MY LUBE TO BE A TASTY TREAT."

BabeLicious lube comes in four tasty flavors: Dulce de Leche, Mojito Peppermint, Pomegranate Vanilla, and Chocolate Orange—while maintaining a glycerin- and paraben-free water-based formula.

What our customers say:

"On a recent trip to the SoHo store, I tried some of the Dulce de Leche on my hand. I was hooked on the smell, and so was he! We went home and tried it—boy, does it make a difference. The smell is strongest, whereas the taste is very light. Perfect! He loved going down on me with it!"

"I WANT A LUBE MADE FROM NATURAL INGREDIENTS."

Botanical, water-based, paraben-free, and infused with aloe, Babeland Naturals Organic Lube (in Naked or Fresh flavors) is compatible with safer-sex barriers and all toy materials. Our lube is never tested on animals, nor are there animal-derived ingredients in it.

What our customers say:

"As someone who gets yeast infections from looking at lube the wrong way, I have been delighted to find that since I made the switch to Naked, I have had a very happy cha cha! It tastes great and smells good too!"

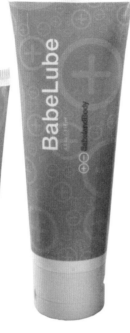
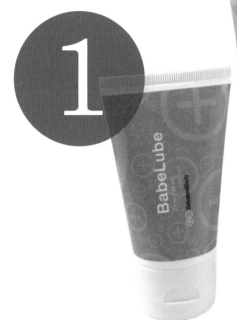
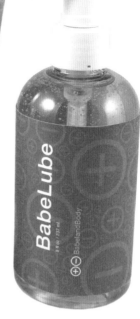

1

BabeLube
BabelandBody

BabeLube
BabelandBody

BabeLube
8 fl oz / 237 ml
BabelandBody

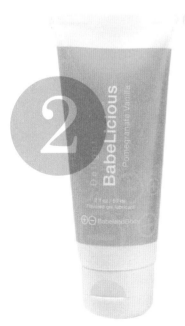
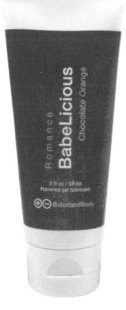

2

Delicate **BabeLicious**
Pomegranate Vanilla
2 fl oz / 59 ml
Flavored gel lubricant
BabelandBody

Romance **BabeLicious**
Chocolate Orange
2 fl oz / 59 ml
Flavored gel lubricant
BabelandBody

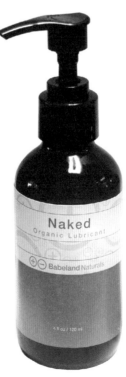
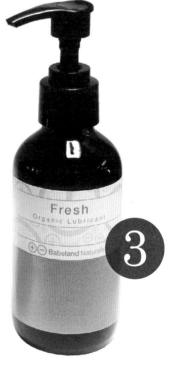

Naked
Organic Lubricant
4 fl oz / 120 ml
Babeland Naturals

Fresh
Organic Lubricant
Babeland Naturals

3

VIBRATORS AND
LABOR-SAVING DEVICES

Some people think of vibrators as the Cliffs Notes of sex—a crutch for cheaters. But guess what? There's no such thing as cheating when you are exploring your body's sexual potential. Hands get tired, they can't reach certain places or bend into every shape, and they don't vibrate like a motor can. (Ditto for tongues.) Vibration brings blood flow, and just plain feels good. Are you cheating if you whip up your cake batter with an electric mixer instead of a spoon? Isn't the cake just as tasty? You see our point. A VIBRATOR CAN BRING ALL KINDS OF NEW POSSIBILITIES AND SENSATIONS. AND YOUR ARM GETS A REST.

CHOOSING A VIBE

How do I pick a vibrator? That's one of the questions we get asked all the time. Often followed by, "What's your favorite?" But that's like asking what your favorite food is. Everyone's different. There are vast and various vibrator choices, which can get overwhelming. But we can help. Let's start with three questions to help steer you toward your first mechanical dream date ...

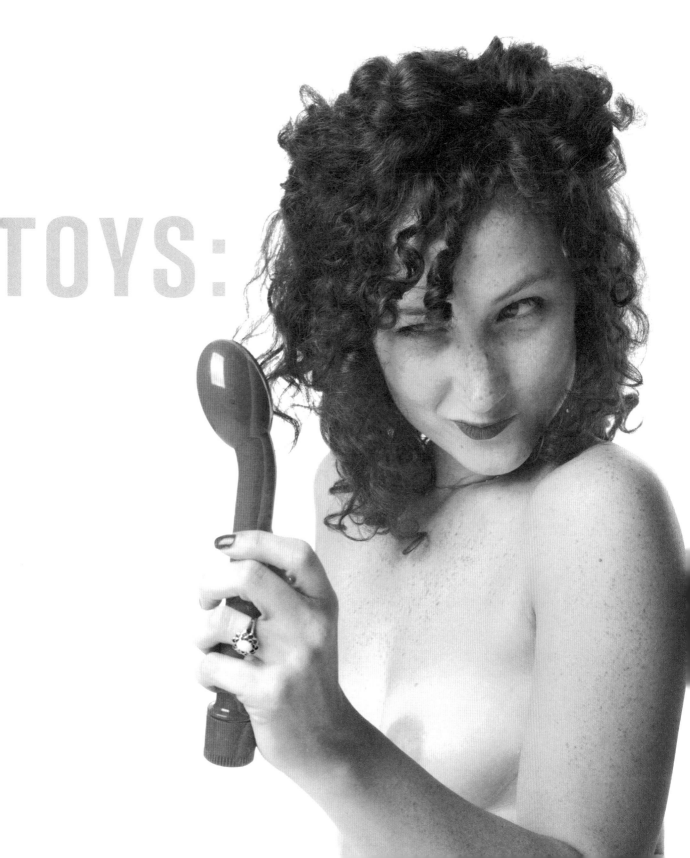

TOYS:

What can your

Question #1
Where do you like your stimulation? Inside or outside?

Most women need clitoral stimulation to get their game on, so our most popular vibes are clit-focused. Others want a vibrator or toy for vaginal penetration, giving a feeling of fullness. Plenty of toy lovers dig both. There are toys that work your clit from the outside and toys that can go inside. And—thanks to the ingenuity of vibrator designers—there are plenty of toys that can do both. If you don't want to make the *Sophie's Choice* of sexual pleasure, a dual-action toy, like the Rabbit Habit (p. 77), which penetrates the pussy and buzzes on the clit, might be your ticket to ride. If you seek anal stimulation, there are toys just for the back door that have a flared base for safe penetration. (You can always buzz around the anal exterior—just don't bring butt bacteria to the vagina.)

Question #2
How strong do you want your vibrations?

Do you work your clit directly and heartily? You might like something strong, like the plug-in vibrators or wand-style vibes with the intensity focused in the tip (p. 74). If you respond to a lighter touch, there are mellower options too, like vibes made with cushier materials. If you're not sure, try one of the many vibes with adjustable speeds and intensities. Then you can experiment and find out which key sparks up your engine.

vibe do for you?

Question #3
What appeals to you?

As in dating, vibrator first impressions and animal attraction do matter. What shapes and colors and textures draw you in? Look at the pictures (p. 75) and see which toys make you curious and excited. We witness this phenomenon in the Babeland stores all the time. A customer will just walk over to a toy with a sparkle in her eye, and her crush begins. This is subjective, unscientific stuff, but it matters. As one customer put it, "As soon as I saw the shiny metal of the Chroma, I fell in love."

And of course ...

There are also matters of price (you may not want to spend a ton on your first vibrator) and portability (are you just keeping it by the bed or taking it on your rock band's tour?), but those three magic questions are the ones to ask yourself first. You can also go to our Web site, www.babeland.com, and check out pictures, descriptions, and even videos to help you make a delightful and satisfying choice.

WHAT DREAM DATES ARE MADE OF: TOY MATERIALS

These are some of the materials commonly used to make vibrators and toys. They transmit vibration differently and need to be cleaned differently. So it helps to know the basics.

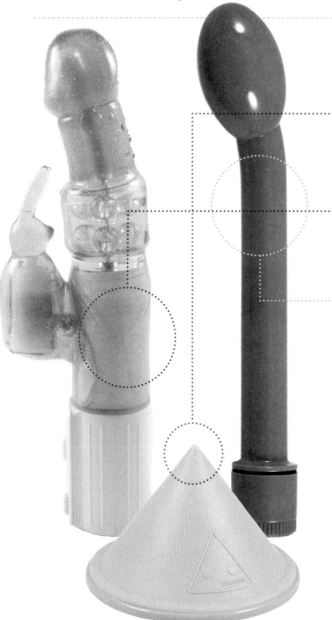

SILICONE

Our favorite material. Soft and pliable. Transmits vibration well, though in a different way than hard surfaces. Agreeable to the body. Pricier. Silicone is completely nonporous and can be cleaned with hot (even boiling) soapy water. Do not use with silicone lube—it might bond to the silicone toy and not come off.

ELASTOMER

A soft plastic without the potentially nasty phthalates. More expensive and worth it.

HARD PLASTIC AND ACRYLIC

Hard to the touch and transmits vibration well. Sometimes slightly noisier (more hard parts can mean more buzz or rattle). Inexpensive. Clean up with plain soap and water. If sharing a hard plastic toy with a partner, slip a condom over it.

VINYL AND JELLY RUBBER: Soft and pliable. The favorite materials of manufacturers because they're incredibly cheap but still soft to the touch. We recommend using a condom even for solo use with these because most soft rubbers contain phthalates. Phthalates are plastic softeners that are around us every day in items like water bottles and shower curtains. Many people question the health impact of the phthalates on our endocrine and reproductive systems. Babeland carries only phthalate-free toys, but they are widely available elsewhere, so we want you to know how to care for them. Clean with soap and water. Definitely use a condom when sharing with partners, since you cannot fully disinfect these materials. Plus the condom makes cleanup a breeze.

CARE AND FEEDING *of your* VIBRATOR

Unless you are really into short-term relationships, here's how to care for your mechanical dream date so the love can last as long as possible.

do

- Store batteries separately. Especially when traveling. You really don't want Homeland Security swarming in to arrest you for a vibrating suitcase. Leaving batteries in can also lead to corrosion. Keep extra batteries handy.

- Wipe your toys clean with warm, soapy water. Don't immerse: use a cloth and air dry.

- Use a condom with soft plastic toys to keep any unsavory chemicals out of your tender places.

- Use condoms on toys you share. The exceptions are silicone toys, which you can boil for ten minutes.

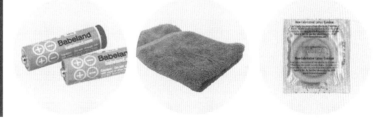

don't

- No backsies-to-frontsies. In other words, no toy goes from your butt to your pussy without a fresh condom on it.

HOW TO VIBRATE WITH PLEASURE

Get ready for your first date with your new purchase. It can go something like this:

1 Just as with old-fashioned manual masturbation, **find a quiet time** in a comfy, private place. Get yourself in the mood in your favorite way: fantasy, porn, erotica, etc.

2 **Find a relaxing position** such as reclining on your back or sitting partway up. Sitting up a bit lets you reach and see better. Have lube nearby and add as needed.

3 **Start your toy** on a lower speed and intensity until you figure out what you like.

4 **Touch your body** in ways that feel good, with your hands or the toy. Run the tip of the vibrator along your body in places like your neck, tummy, and nipples.

5 When you're ready to up the ante, bring the vibrator to your vulva and **start exploring** and experimenting. Press the tip or the side of the vibe against different parts: the mons, the outer labia, the perineum, the vaginal opening. Try different kinds of pressure and different speeds. Notice when your body says, "Yes, more of that," or "No, that's too much," or "Buzzing here is annoying or boring." Touch the tip of the vibrator near the clit, then over the hood, before you touch it directly. Your clit has so many nerves—all rigged to give you pleasure—that it will likely be the focus of your vibrator play. Get your clit excited, then back off. Then buzz on or near it again.

What do I actually DO a vibrator when I get

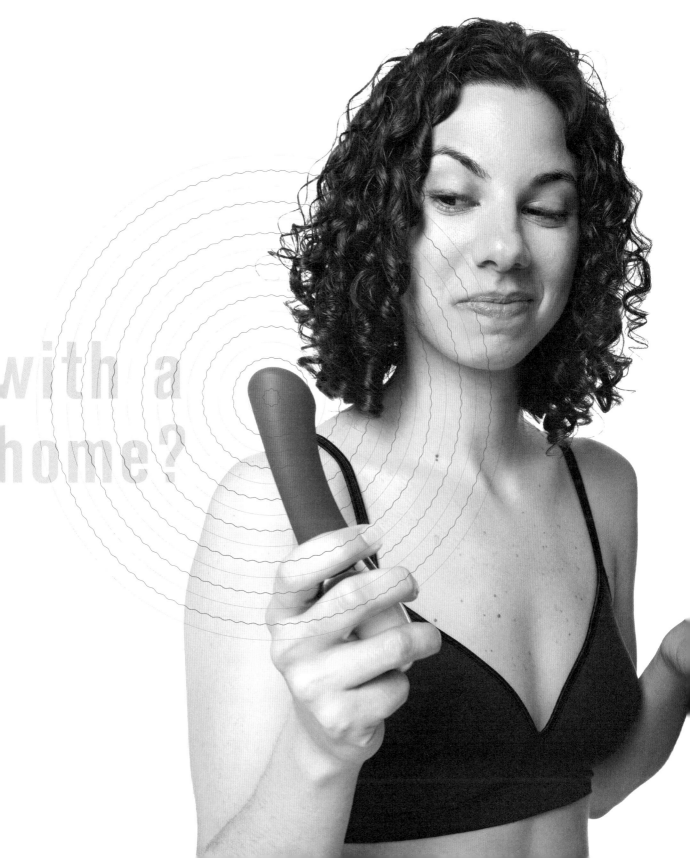

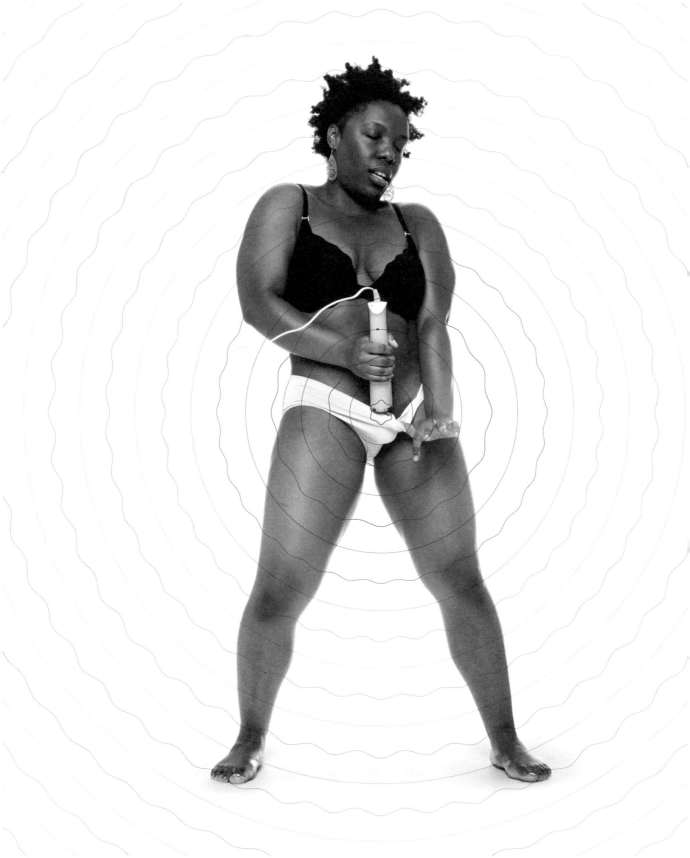

VARY YOUR VIBE

Keep things interesting by trying these exercises.

1 The Sexy Spiral

Use the tip of your buzzing vibrator to slowly draw a circle the width of your whole vulva. Then keep tracing smaller and smaller circles within that one, spiraling in toward the clit. As you get closer to your clit epicenter, stop and play wherever it feels great. You can do it in reverse or start over. You're the maestro.

2 The Extra Gentle Vibe

If the vibration is just too intense, try putting a blanket or a pillow between you and the vibe.

3 Be on Your Back, on Top, or on Your Side

As with manual masturbation, you can try different positions, such as lying on your stomach with the vibe under you. You can control the movements with your pelvis or hand or both. Or, if you are on your back, compare having your legs apart to keeping your feet together and knees apart.

4 Bring In the Other Hand

Add your free hand to the playground. Caress your breasts. Or you can buzz your clit with the right hand while inserting fingers from your left hand into your pussy. Added bonus: if you come, you'll feel pelvic spasms around your inserted fingers.

{ Q & A }

PULSATING CONCERNS

{Q} "Will a vibrator make me numb?"

{A} A vibrator will not damage the nerve endings on your clit or anywhere on your V. After a long or intense roll in the mechanical hay, a vibrator can tire out the nerves, making them feel numb temporarily—much like your hand might feel numb after writing for a long time. The feeling will come back 100 percent. Just take a break. Also be aware of the different kinds of vibration out there. Some people don't like really fast and steady vibration. They feel like it annoys and desensitizes more than it stimulates. They prefer vibration that's more low-pitched and rumbly. We call this the "buzzy vs. thumpy" option. And there are way more than two options. There are vibrators that move and oscillate at all kinds of intensities and speeds. This is just another matter of taste.

{Q} "How often do I need to buy a new vibe?"

{A} These are hard times for both our wallets and for Mother Earth. But vibrators, by their very nature, shake and rattle and eventually tire themselves out. And then they are landfill fodder. So once you know what kind of vibe you like, it pays to invest in a more expensive one that will last longer. This is also a good reason to get an electric vibe with a cord, or a rechargeable vibe (which recharges like a cell phone). They last a really long time and don't need batteries. If your favorite vibe takes batteries, try rechargeable batteries. And though most sex toys are plastic, we also sell ones that are made of metal, glass, and even wood.

{Q} "Can I get addicted?"

{A} We hear this question a lot. And that's too bad. It confirms an idea floating around in our culture that getting off is dangerous and a woman might just be having too much pleasure. We certainly don't think masturbation is a bad habit like cocaine or drunk-texting or high-stakes roulette. Jilling off makes you more alert and alive. What the asker often means is, "Will a vibrator be the only thing that can make me come and then I'll be ruined for anything else?"

The answer is still no. You might get into a sexual rut, where you've found a surefire way to give yourself an orgasm (and, by the way, congratulations for that). But when you only get off that one way, it starts to have about as much meaning and excitement as brushing your teeth. A lot of the joy of sexual pleasure is discovering new things and feeling new ways. So try broadening your horizons with a new technique. Stash the toy in a drawer for a while. Try a different one. Take a break. It'll always be there later when you need it.

{Q} "My vibrator makes my partner feel inadequate."

{A} To your lover, and particularly to guys, who have generally been left out of the vibrator revolution, a vibrator can seem like competition. It's a common mistake to judge one's sexual prowess by what one can deliver unaided. If you're bringing toys to bed for the first time, and you think your partner may feel threatened by one that looks like a penis, introduce vibes that look more like a friendly toy—perhaps a round, eggy one. Introduce a toy into your partner sex, and show your lover what you like to do with it, which will probably turn both of you on. Teach your partner how to take control and use it on you. Add it to sex, like buzzing your clit while you are being entered from behind. By then your sweetheart will probably understand that your vibe adds fun and pleasure, and everybody wins. Sometime when you are not having hot vibey sex with your partner, remind Mr. Boyfriend or Ms. Girlfriend that you find them foxy, and that your vibe can't make out, cuddle, or tell a good story like they can.

{Q} "I like something inside me though."

{A} If the feeling of penetration and being "filled up" are essential turn-ons for you, you might want to jill yourself off with a dildo. Many wand-shaped vibrators like the beloved Rabbit Habit combine vibration with penetration. Great. But sometimes you just want something smooth and delicious to stimulate that hungry puss. Fingers can only do so much. And if you are fingering yourself, you might put out your elbow with the tricky angle. Dildos are also fine tools for reaching the G-spot or prostate—many are designed and angled just for that purpose. If you are interested in dildoing up yourself, think about some of the following questions: Is it more exciting to me if it looks like a cock? If so, do I want it to have balls too? Am I more interested in a sleek shape that gets the job done? Do I want it to be solid? (We sell dils made of glass or steel that are beautiful!) Or do I prefer it more soft and supple? Silicone and elastomer have more give—like flesh. It helps to see and touch dildos in person and see what makes your eyes (and nether places) light up. Using a dildo with a condom makes for easy cleanup and safer sharing. And lube is handy to have around if you need it. (See also The Satisfied Customer: Dildos, p. 212.)

SATISFIED CUSTOMER

The

⊕⊖

{THE VIBE GUIDE}

Need a little help deciding which vibrator to buy? The truly amazing array of styles, sizes, and materials can be both inspiring and a little daunting. Whether you're shopping for yourself or a partner, here are some common requests we hear. They will help cut through the information overload and guarantee a delightful spin with your new toy. Plus, reviews from the toughest critics out there: our customers.

"I WANT A VIBE FOR CLITORAL STIMULATION."

Just about anything that vibrates feels good on or around the clitoris. Smaller clit vibes like the Laya Spot are easy to use, and stronger vibes like the Hitachi (shown with the G-whiz attachment) will help you come quickly.

What our customers say:

"I love my Laya Spot, and so does my boyfriend. I tried it on him one time during a blow job, and I actually ended up having to buy one for him too because I'd always catch him with it!"

"Unbelievable. The Hitachi Wand is my sex toy. It is amazing that I can climax within five minutes with this toy. Damn, damn, damn."

"I WANT A VIBE THAT WILL PUT ME IN TOUCH WITH MY G-SPOT."

The Orchid G wins rave reviews, as does the silicone Gigi vibrator. Look for vibes with a curve toward the tip.

What our customers say:

"I've had the Orchid G for about a year and have never regretted it! I found my G-spot and have even ejaculated a few times—which I had never done before!"

"Nothing can describe the feelings I get from the Gigi. If this toy could slap me and call me a dirty slut, I'd let it!"

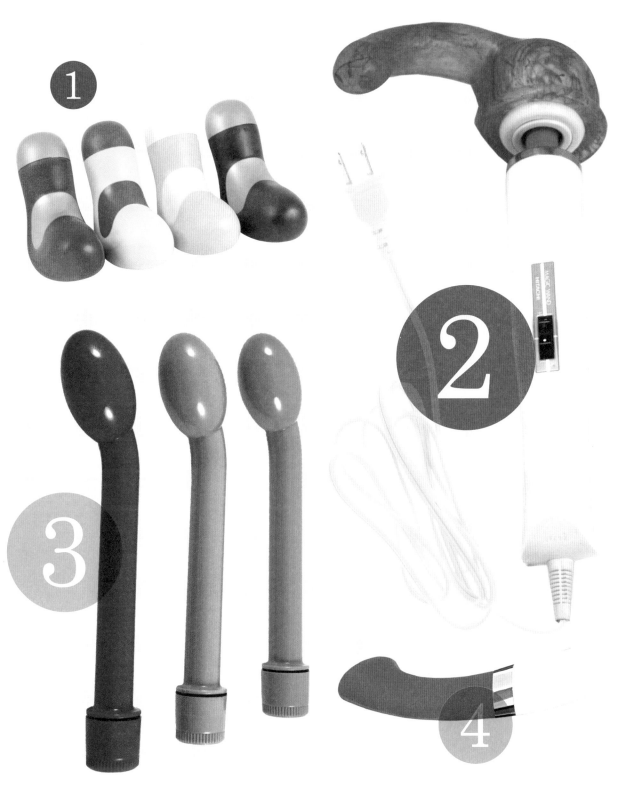

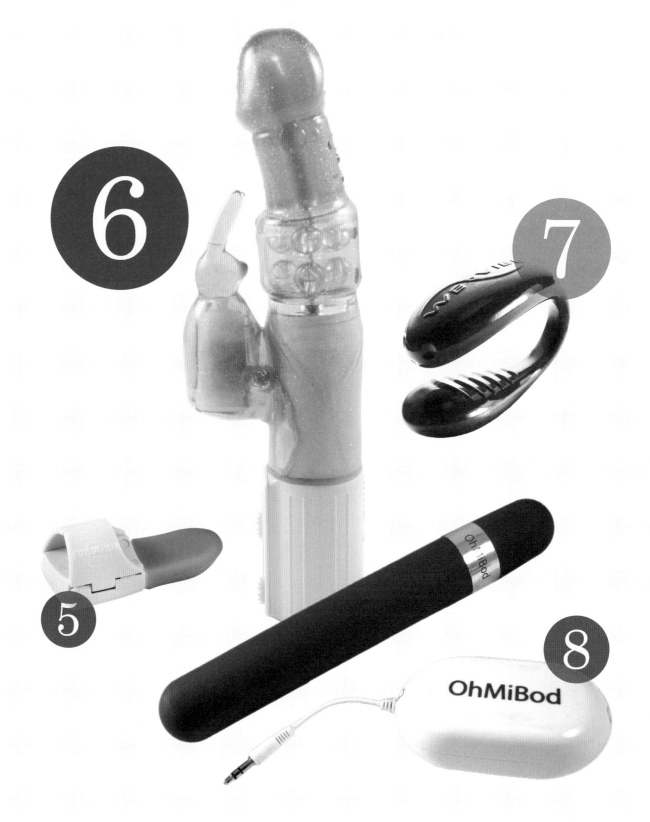

⑤

"I'M LOOKING FOR A VIBRATOR TO GIVE MY HAND A LITTLE EXTRA OOMPH."

The Fukuoku is a tiny vibrator that slides right over your finger. It is great for masturbation. You can also have your partner wear one to stimulate your clit in a variety of positions.

What our customers say:

"Recently, I decided it might not be a bad idea to take a more digital approach to pleasure. I have enjoyed the added intimacy of feeling myself with my fingers. The Fukuoku has helped me to better learn my own unique anatomy—from texture and location to size."

⑥

"I WOULD LIKE A VIBE THAT CAN BE USED ON MY CLIT AND MY G-SPOT."

For a vibe that stimulates both pleasure points at once, try the international vibrating celebrity: Rabbit Habit.

What our customers say:

"My Rabbit is great! It sends me into multiple orgasms just about every time I use it. I like to start with just the rabbit ears on my clit and then insert so the rotating balls can join in and take me over the edge!"

⑦

"I WANT A VIBE I CAN USE HANDS-FREE WITH MY PARTNER."

Try the We Vibe, truly a standout in a sea of couple's toys. We know, because we've seen 'em all. This silicone two-speed vibrator is completely waterproof, easy to clean, rechargeable, and a dream come true.

What our customers say:

"As far as I'm concerned, the We Vibe is the greatest invention since electricity. The We Vibe has already given me weeks worth of ecstasy solo, and when I used it during sex, I thought I was going to die of pleasure. My boyfriend loved it too."

⑧

"I WANT A VIBRATOR WITH A SOUNDTRACK."

Plug into pleasures as diverse as your playlist with the tech-savvy Freestyle by OhMiBod. This velvety-soft toy vibrates to match your music, beat for beat—wirelessly!

What our customers say:

"This product really does work perfectly with music. I've used it with my iPod and with my laptop during a video chat with my partner for a completely amazing enhanced phone-sex experience! It was absolutely fabulous!"

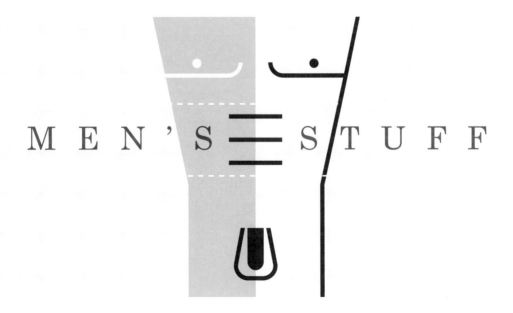

CHAPTER 3

MEN'S STUFF

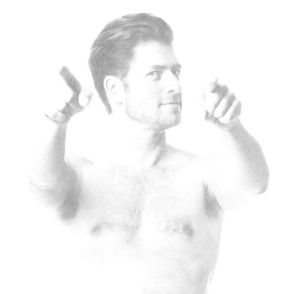

GETTING TO

If your partner is a guy, it's gonna help to know how his equipment works. Guys have an enviable level of familiarity with their genitals. How could they not? Penises hang outside the body and demand interaction. Think about it: a man sees and touches his penis every time he pees. He aims, shoots, and shakes off in a little ritual that's been going on a half-dozen

KNOW HIM

times per day since late toddlerhood. So guys become very comfortable touching themselves. We want to help you catch up by offering a crash course in Penis-ology 101. The more you know about your guy's package, the better you can work it. Much like the men you love, those packages are more complex and nuanced than they might first appear. Behold.

THE PENIS AND FRIENDS

The Anatomy of Male Pleasure

Ah, the penis. Volumes have been written on it, from *Moby Dick* to *Portnoy's Complaint*. But for his maximum enjoyment, this is all the required reading you need.

EXTERNAL { Fig. A }:

1. PENIS

Often considered the star of the sex show, the penis contains neither bones nor muscle. Increased blood flow to erectile tissue is what makes the penis stand up and perform. The penis is the male version of the clitoris—both have a glans (a head) and a shaft. And like the clitoris, you cannot see the whole unit. The penis has a base, rooted inches deeper in the pelvic cavity, where you can still stimulate it.

2. GLANS (HEAD)

This is the tip. The most sensitive part of the penis, the glans has the most nerves. (The glans of the clit has even more—not that it's a competition.) An uncircumcised fella will have a more sensitive glans because his foreskin protects it from the elements and keeps it moist with mucus. And this is a great thing! It means your every touch will feel amazing. Cut or uncut, treat the glans like you'd treat your clit—with lots of loving attention. Maybe start out with gentle swirly licks, increasing the pressure and roughness until the owner declares you Queen of the Universe.

3. CORONAL RIDGE

The ridge around the base of the glans. This is the more sensitive part of the already sensitive glans. "Corona" means "crown" (not "beer"), so treat this ridge with the loving care a king would give his crown. You can trace circles around the corona with your tongue or your lubed finger. All hail!

4. URETHRAL OPENING

The pee hole in the tip of the glans. It's where both urine and semen come out—but never at the same time. It's sensitive, so some guys find it a source of pleasure and like it touched (a little sucking, a little tongue flicker). Other dudes want you to keep the heck off it. Depends on the owner.

5. FRENULUM

You know what they say: Keep your friends close and your frenulum closer. The frenulum is a little piece of skin, almost like a bit of webbing, where the shaft meets the glans on the underside. On some men, that flap of skin was partially or completely removed during circumcision. But the bundle of nerves remains, making it arguably the most sensitive spot on the penis. A magical wonder-spot. Guys generally love it when you flick and flutter the tip of

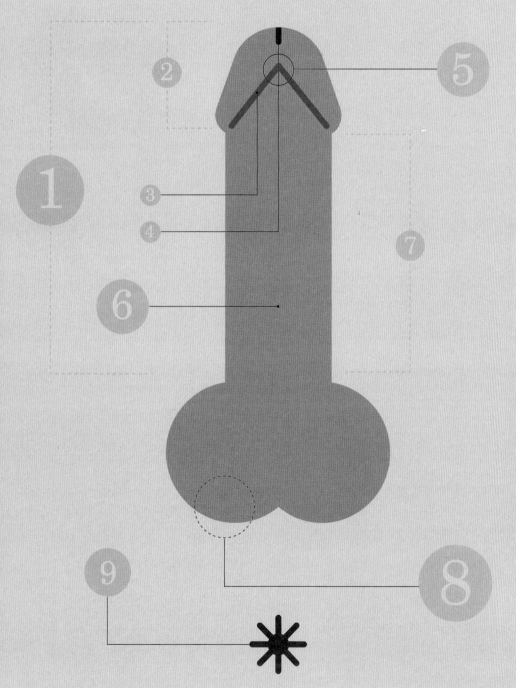

{ Fig. A }
EXTERNAL VIEW

your tongue over the frenulum during a BJ. If you're
working with your hands, give it a little massage
with one or both of your lubed-up thumbs.

6. RAPHE

Pronounced "RAY-fee." The ridge that runs along
the underside of a man's package from the frenulum,
down the shaft, along the scrotum, and to the anus.
Can be extra sensitive. You can think of it as the
seam that nature sewed when the body developed
into a male instead of a female. In fact, "raphe" is
from the Greek word for "seam."

7. SHAFT

The part of the penis that grows the most during arousal. Think of it as the trunk of his tree.
Size-wise, erections are the great equalizer in that
smaller guys often get way bigger when aroused,
and bigger dudes often grow just a little when
aroused. Is your guy a "grower" or a "show-er"?
The skin over the shaft is somewhat loose, so you
can slide it up and down over the shaft, which feels
good—especially with lube. Like the shaft of your
clit, the shaft of his cock enjoys a good stroking to
get the whole area worked up.

8. SCROTUM

The sac of skin that holds the testicles. It's equivalent to the labia in women. The scrotum pulls the
testicles up into the body for warmth or lets them
dangle to cool off. Many men enjoy caressing, squeezing, and even pulling on the scrotum when aroused.
Ask first, however. Your sweetie might be ticklish.

9. ANUS

The opening that leads to the rectum and then the
colon. (See also His Butt, p. 86.)

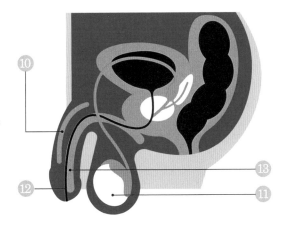

{ FIG. B } INTERNAL VIEW

FORESKIN *(not shown)*

All males are born with a retractable sheath of
skin that protects the glans like a cozy turtleneck
sweater. Many American baby boys get circumcised,
a procedure in which the foreskin is removed. It's
more of a cultural tradition than a medical neces-
sity. But uncut penises are coming back into style,
so don't be surprised to find that your lover still has
his foreskin. If that is the case, you can incorporate
the foreskin into moves you already know. The loose
extra skin can slide up and down the shaft, making
hand jobs a breeze. If you want to get oral on him,
slide the foreskin down toward the base to access
and enjoy his extra sensitive glans.

INTERNAL { Fig. B }:

10. CORPORA CAVERNOSA

The phrase means "cavelike bodies" and refers to
the two long cylinders of spongy erectile tissue that

make the penis grow when they fill with blood (they actually hold 90 percent of the blood that flows into the cock when it's hard). These are analogous to the clitoral legs in women. And like the clitoral legs, they are loaded with nerve endings and love to be stroked and stimulated.

11. TESTICLES

A.k.a. "fantas-ticles," these guys are main players in the manufacture of sperm and testosterone. They can be as small as grapes or as big as eggs. One can hang lower than the other. The testicles are extremely sensitive to pain, as everyone who has ever heard of them knows. So handle with care.

12. URETHRA

As in women, this is the tube leading out from the bladder. Urine and semen are both expelled out the urethra. In a stroke of design genius, the muscles around the opening of the bladder close the gates when a guy is turned on, preventing pee and semen from flowing through the urethra at the same time. This is why a guy with a morning hard-on has a tough time letting loose his morning pee. And why you can rest assured that a man with a hard-on cannot pee on you.

13. CORPUS SPONGIOSUM (URETHRAL SPONGE)

A cylinder of spongy tissue that surrounds the urethra (picture bubble wrap around a straw). Fills up with blood when aroused. Along with the corpora cavernosa, the corpus spongiosum puts the "erect" in "erection." Note: it doesn't get as hard as the rest of the shaft. It stays spongy so that the urethra doesn't get squeezed shut, which would block the exit for the semen.

DON'T FORGET HIS NIPS!

Your guy's nipples can be just as sensitive as a woman's. Watch and see if they get darker or erect during arousal. Touch and nibble on them to get his motor running, or maybe even give nipple clamps a try. These small pinching clips for the nips are an equal opportunity sex toy that both partners may enjoy.

Kissing, touching, and licking the nipple can be as hot for him as it is for you.

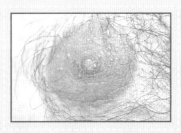

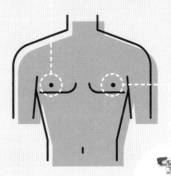

To find out more about nipple clamps, see p. 136.

To find out more about nipple clamps, see p. 136.

HIS BUTT
Backdoor Fun

Think of all the wonderful things that come through the backdoor of your house—special deliveries, close friends. His anatomical back door enjoys special deliveries and the love of close friends too. While a guy has the same kind of perineum, rectum, super sensitive nerve endings, and sphincters as a woman, the prostate makes backdoor visits even more exciting for him. You can reach places he can't, and you can make his world explode. What a gift!

1. PERINEUM
A.k.a. the "taint" (just remember: "T'aint nice to ignore it"). The bridge of smooth skin between the scrotum and the anus. As with women, the perineum is sensitive and gets flushed and excited during sex play. The male perineum is a great place to feel and stimulate the root of the penis, massaging it from the outside.

2. RECTUM
Rectal tissue is very delicate and has a subtle S-curve in shape, which can matter when probing within. The rectum tips slightly toward the belly side, and you reach the prostate gland through the belly-side wall of the rectum, so it's good to point your fingers and toys at that angle.

3. INTERNAL SPHINCTER MUSCLE
A ring-shaped muscle that forms the inner gateway to and from the rectum. It cannot be consciously tightened or relaxed. When poop comes down the chute to be expelled, the pressure on the internal sphincter signals that it's time to find a loo. The internal sphincter will shut tightly and register pain if anyone tries to storm (or assertively poke) the gate. So think of the internal sphincter as a very serious bouncer that will only let you into the VIP Club if you are really sweet and patient and smooth the way with lots of lube.

4. OUTER SPHINCTER MUSCLE
A ring-shaped muscle that forms the outer gateway to and from the rectum. This is more under the owner's control and command, allowing him (or her) to poop at the right time and place. With patience, communication, and lube, this muscle will open and welcome penetration. Sphincters work the same way in both guys and dolls.

5. PROSTATE
Just under the bladder. Forms a doughnut around the urethra. The prostate makes 30 percent of the ejaculatory fluid that carries and nourishes the sperm. When a guy is excited, his prostate responds well to rhythmic stimulation. Some men can orgasm from prostate stimulation alone. But it's also

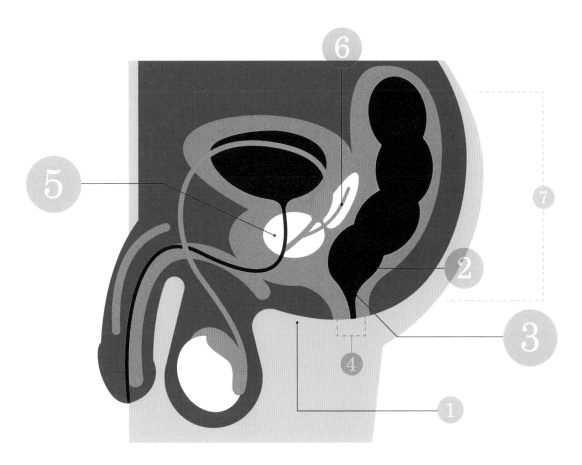

one of the reasons that guys like a finger or two up the bum when they are excited. Curve your finger toward his belly about two inches in, and there's the jackpot. The prostate is similar to the G-spot in women.

6. SEMINAL VESICLES

Small structures that attach to the prostate and connect to the urethra. They manufacture 70 percent of the fluid that becomes semen.

7. PC MUSCLE

Like the PC muscle in women, this "floor" of muscle stretches from the tailbone to the pelvic bone and holds up the internal organs. This muscle also helps control the elimination of pee and poop. Its sexier task is holding the tension that builds up during sex play and gets released with orgasm.

THE BASIC ORDER OF OPERATIONS: THE MALE SEXUAL RESPONSE

We encourage our female customers to be responsible for their orgasms—and to lovingly, patiently seek out the big O if it's been elusive. Our advice for men (and their partners) is almost the opposite: Lovingly, patiently let go of the big O as the centerpiece of your sex play. We think orgasms are great, but it's easy to fall into the habit of making your fella's explosion the goal, and then ta-da! You're both done. It's understandable, because when he shoots, it can be like a dramatic finale. But don't let the finale take over the whole opera. This can leave a gal frustrated. This can make a guy feel pressured.

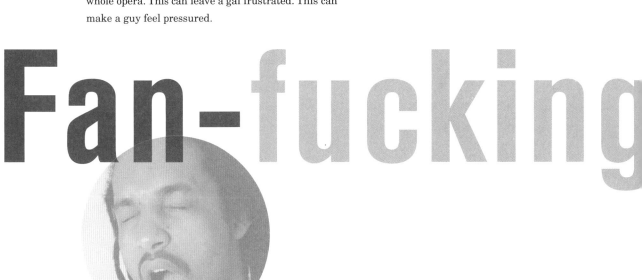

Fan-fucking

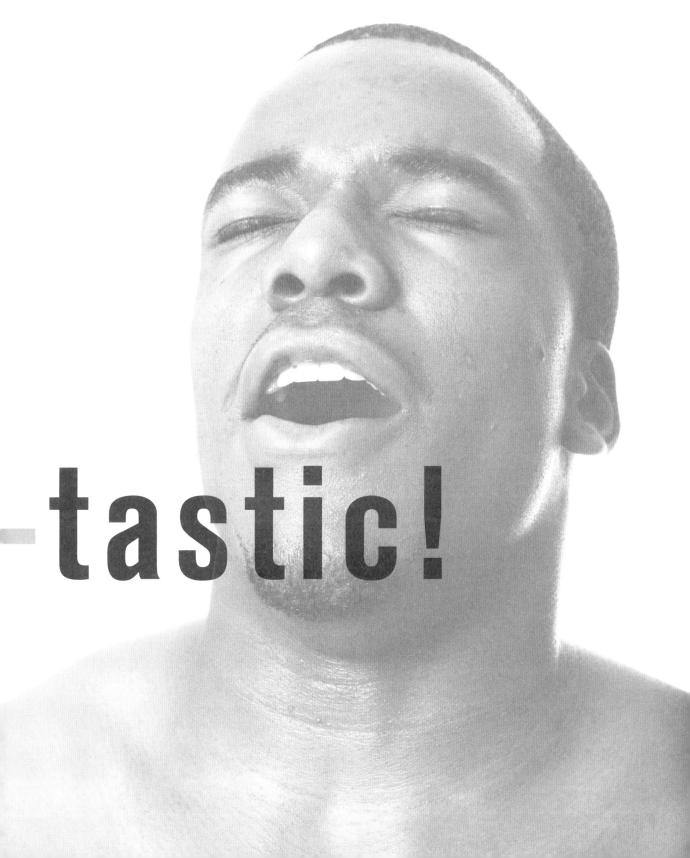

-tastic!

Stages of
HIS ORGASM

These are four stages on a typical male sex journey, but he doesn't have to follow this route directly. He can go from stage one to two, back to one, then two to three to two. And of course the stages overlap. These are just some signposts to look for along the way.

Stage One: Arousal

As he gets excited from kissing or seeing something provocative or getting touched, his heartbeat speeds up and his blood flow increases, sending blood to the lips, cheeks, and whole pelvic area. He might feel warmth all over and his skin may be flushed. Tension builds up in his muscles. An erection may begin or get all the way there, and his nipples might get hard too. There's an increased sensitivity to touch everywhere, and decreased sensitivity to pain. His scrotum starts to contract, and the testicles elevate.

Stage Two: Plateau

All of the above changes continue. His penis gets bigger and more rigid. In fact, the corpora cavernosa expand and squeeze shut the veins that would normally carry blood out of the penis—thus ensuring a hard hard-on. His tissues are engorged throughout the whole package and anus. A little bit of clear glandular fluid comes out the tip of the penis (a.k.a. "pre-come"). There might be a few sperm in the drop of pre-come, but it mainly serves as extra lube. His muscle tension builds further. The scrotum and testicles pull up in preparation for ejaculation. You can pull down on the scrotum (with permission!) and encourage steady, deep breathing to draw out this stage.

Stage Three: Climax

His heart rate and breathing intensify. There's a moment when he gives up conscious control of his body and lets the orgasm take over. At this stage, there's often a feeling of wild abandon. Muscle contractions radiate from the penis and the pelvic floor—and can take place anywhere on the body. His hands or face or feet may even twitch. The muscle spasms release tension and send blood out of the pelvic zip code. The muscles around the opening of the bladder clench. The testicles and prostate send their cocktail of sperm and fluid out the urethra. The brain releases feel-good neurochemicals.

Stage Four: Resolution

His breathing and blood flow return to normal. The penis and other parts return to their everyday shape and color. If there was no climax, it can take longer for the body to return to its resting state. There can even be a dull ache in the testicles (a.k.a. "blue balls"), which is harmless and temporary.

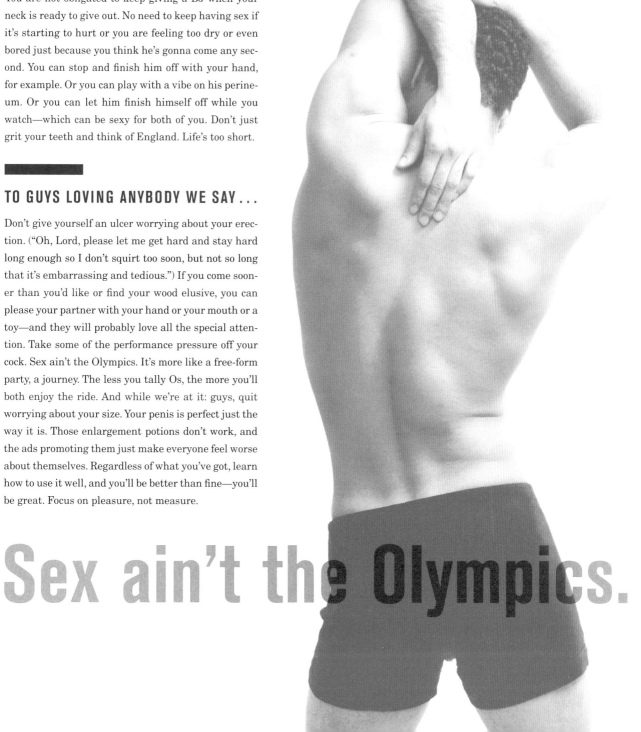

TO CHICKS LOVING GUYS WE SAY...

You are not obligated to keep giving a BJ when your neck is ready to give out. No need to keep having sex if it's starting to hurt or you are feeling too dry or even bored just because you think he's gonna come any second. You can stop and finish him off with your hand, for example. Or you can play with a vibe on his perineum. Or you can let him finish himself off while you watch—which can be sexy for both of you. Don't just grit your teeth and think of England. Life's too short.

TO GUYS LOVING ANYBODY WE SAY...

Don't give yourself an ulcer worrying about your erection. ("Oh, Lord, please let me get hard and stay hard long enough so I don't squirt too soon, but not so long that it's embarrassing and tedious.") If you come sooner than you'd like or find your wood elusive, you can please your partner with your hand or your mouth or a toy—and they will probably love all the special attention. Take some of the performance pressure off your cock. Sex ain't the Olympics. It's more like a free-form party, a journey. The less you tally Os, the more you'll both enjoy the ride. And while we're at it: guys, quit worrying about your size. Your penis is perfect just the way it is. Those enlargement potions don't work, and the ads promoting them just make everyone feel worse about themselves. Regardless of what you've got, learn how to use it well, and you'll be better than fine—you'll be great. Focus on pleasure, not measure.

Sex ain't the Olympics.

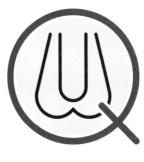

{ Q & A }

THROBBING CONCERNS

{Q} "What's the difference between orgasm and ejaculation?"

{A} Like peanut butter and jelly, orgasm and ejaculation are two different things that go great together. Coming and shooting are separate events triggered by two separate sets of nerves and muscles. Ejaculation happens when the muscles around the prostate gland contract, which releases fluid. Guys can feel that "thar-she-blows, I'm coming" sensation. (Doctors call it "ejaculatory inevitability.") Orgasm is the set of rhythmic muscular contractions throughout the penis and beyond. It's possible to squirt before you orgasm. And it's possible to orgasm without squirting. There are techniques involving slow, controlled breathing and concentration that allow men to separate the two happy events. Without ejaculation, it's theoretically easier to have multiple orgasms and go all night. One benefit of ejaculation is that regularly cleaning out the pipes is good for long-term prostate health.

{Q} "Can men have multiple orgasms?"

{A} Yes, but not as easily as women have them. Men generally need recovery time after an orgasm. But some men (usually young men) have very short recovery periods after an O, so they can do it again and again. Other men have trained themselves to come without ejaculating—which also makes for shorter recovery time.

{Q} "My guy has trouble getting (and staying) hard."

{A} This happens to all men at some point. Stress, smoking, boozing, fatigue, some medications (like commonly prescribed SSRI-inhibiting antidepressants), and certain medical conditions are common reasons. It probably has nothing to do with his desire for you, so don't take it personally. At all. It sounds like a nice opportunity to ask for a luxurious round of oral pleasure. Enjoy it as long as you want. If his jaw gets tired, bust out the vibrator. This is what we mean by getting away from goal-oriented ejacu-centric sex. That said, if he has an ongoing problem getting an erection, there could be a bigger health issue like diabetes or circulation problems. Or something as simple as aging. For these cases of medical erectile dysfunction (E.D.), see a doctor. While we're not fans of turning to pharmaceuticals first, sometimes they're a big help. Does your sweetie get morning boners? If he does, then the equipment is working—just not on demand. In that case, we recommend giving partner sex and even masturbation a rest for a few days or longer so your mind and body can hit the reset button and get back in sync.

{Q} "How do I help my boyfriend with his premature ejaculation?"

{A} For starters, be careful about calling it that—the term implies there's a "mature" or right time to ejaculate. There are no set rules about how long sex should take. Do you think it's "premature" because he comes before you get a chance to? We understand that'd be frustrating. But if you know that's your honey's pattern, then negotiate a way to get you off sooner—maybe from oral or manual stimulation—even before his cock goes inside you. If you want to work on slowing down and delaying his money shot, there's a simple exercise he can try. On his own time, he might try masturbating right up to that "ejaculatory inevitability." Then he should pause all movement—maybe take a few deep breaths—until the excitement ebbs a bit. He could repeat this a couple of times until he is ready to come by choice. After practice at home, he can try this same exercise during sex with you. He might also try a cock ring, which helps keep blood in the penis longer. Even a condom will help—it restricts blood flow at the base. But we think it's best to avoid products like numbing creams (or disassociating through mental tricks like reciting the Constitution). It's much nicer to keep your mind and body in the game—not out of it.

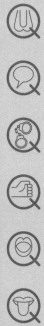

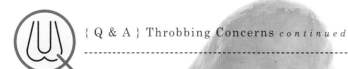
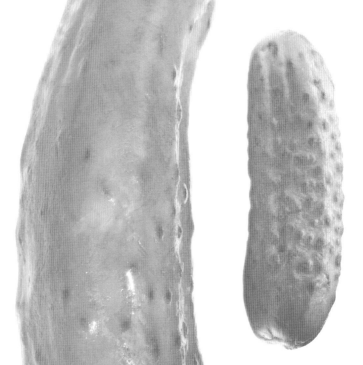

{ Q }

"What's the deal with dick size?"

{ A } People make a big thing (ahem) about penis size. Clearly it's an issue, or our spam filters wouldn't be clogged with subject lines like "Turn your garden snake into an anaconda" and "Get a giant knob of steel." We believe strongly that it's not the size of the ship but the motion of the ocean that matters. For certain folks, a super big penis is something of a fetish, like the way some guys like super big breasts. But for most of us, it's not that important. Remember that both the vagina and rectum are more like envelopes than tunnels—you don't need a lot of penis to make them feel full and good. But there are times and positions when a penis can feel "loose" in your V. Maybe you are really lubed up. Maybe when you are very turned on, your "vaginal ballooning" is in full effect. Doggy style and rear-entry positions will feel tighter. If you crave that "stuffed" feeling, a guy can wrap his hand around his dick in a way that lets him slide in some fingers too.

{Q} "What is the average penis length?"

{A} Measuring from the base of the shaft to the tip, the average length at rest is about three inches. Erect? About five inches. Some guys are "growers" not "show-ers," meaning they start on the small side but gain many inches when hard. (Boner fact: an erect penis can hold as much as eight times the amount of blood in a resting penis.) Other guys are big when flaccid and don't get much bigger when erect.

{Q} "My boyfriend has a third leg, I swear. How do I manage?"

{A} Though easy on the eyes, a very large cock has its down sides. Use your hands a lot during a bonus-size blow job. If the penis is really big, it can bump the cervix during sex, and that can hurt (or just be annoying). If his manhood is monstrous, ask him to take extra care with rear-entry positions—he can play with the angle or just not push all the way in. Take your time and use lots of lube.

{Q} "My guy's penis is a funny color."

{A} Penises, like all the other parts of the body, come in a million different shapes, shades, and styles. That's what makes us all unique. Maybe your lover's penis is darker-skinned than the rest of his body. Maybe he even has a dark ring around his penis. Both are common and perfectly fine.

{Q} "I just encountered my first curved penis. How normal is this?"

{A} An estimated 5 percent of men have some degree of bend or curve in their penises. In most cases, a curved penis is not cause for concern. You do all the usual stuff with a curved penis. It feels the same and works the same. You might have lucked out and found a partner with a built-in G-spot massager! Try different positions that help him hit your sweet spot, wherever it is.

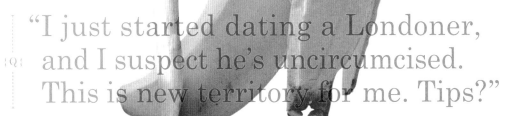

"I just started dating a Londoner, and I suspect he's uncircumcised. This is new territory for me. Tips?"

The foreskin might be your new best friend. If you've never seen one, it's like a legwarmer (ha—third legwarmer) that covers the head of the penis. Or since he's British, we'll call it his tea cozy. The foreskin is sensitive and lined with a mucus membrane. It keeps the head sensitive and more lubed than the glans of a circumcised fellow. Some tips for handling his tea cozy:

• Since the head of his dick is probably more sensitive, start out extra gently with your manual and oral maneuvers—at least with direct contact on the glans. The foreskin corresponds to the clitoral hood on a woman. Think how exposed your clit can feel when it comes out from under its hood.

• Use the foreskin to your advantage—you can slide it up and down as a hand-job helper.

• Be sure to pull the foreskin back when putting on a condom.

• Ask your lover to guide you—even demonstrate his favorite hand techniques. Watch his signals as you play—and check in by asking—to make sure your moves are well received.

"I find my boyfriend's morning wood a big turn-on, but he shoos me away when I try to climb aboard."

{Q}

{A} It certainly is nice to wake up and see his flag waving a "good morning" to ya. But wake-up wood is more of a mechanical test run. It doesn't automatically include desire. So treat his morning boner as if you are starting from a limp penis. Coax and fondle it (and its owner) before getting permission to climb aboard. Your man might very well have a full bladder that he'll want to empty first (which could take a minute, since a hard-on means the urethra is ready for semen, not urine, to exit). There are also guys who like the heightened feeling of sex with some extra bladder pressure. (Some women do too.)

"Why do men constantly touch their penises? I mean, really?"

{Q}

{A} We are not psychologists, but we can certainly observe and opine here. Because the penis hangs outside the body, men feel a combination of pride and vulnerability. The quick gesture of front-end alignment is soothing and says, "Still there and ticking? Check." Plus, ball skin can stick to thigh skin and make a guy feel like he needs to get unstuck.

"What's in semen?"

{Q}

{A} Semen is mostly glandular fluid that helps keep the sperm alive and happy. A small amount of the male cocktail is actual swimming sperm from the testicles. The prostate kicks in 15 to 30 percent of the recipe, and the seminal vesicles squirt in 70 percent of the total load. It's all harmless to swallow if you want to—though some people get a slightly upset stomach from it. There's zinc in semen—which is good for you but can taste icky. There's magnesium, which gives the salty flavor. There's also some fructose and glucose, which are sweet. And while we're on the topic, here's what you can expect in a dose: though porn movies make ejaculation look like a geyser at Yellowstone Park, the average output of semen is about a teaspoon or less.

"Why does semen smell like bleach?"

{Q}

{A} Sperm and testicular fluid are actually odorless. But the contributions from the seminal vesicles and the prostate create the odor. The prostate releases a chemical aptly called "spermine" that causes the Clorox-y smell. Spermine is also an irritant if it gets in your eye—it can sting or cause an infection.

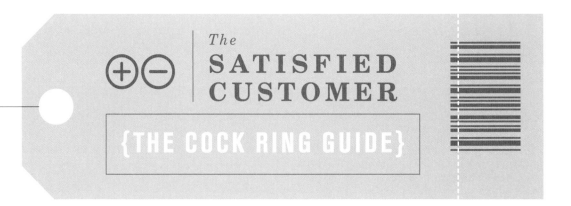

The

SATISFIED
CUSTOMER

{THE COCK RING GUIDE}

Cock rings will help heighten a man's sensitivity and help keep him hard longer by playing with dick circulation in a way that can feel good. The vessels that send blood into the dick are embedded more deeply inside the shaft than the ones that pump blood back out. Because of this plumbing arrangement, cock rings–which squeeze the outer surface of the penis–let blood in but slow it from pumping out. Thanks, Mother Nature! Basically, it's a strap of leather or rubber (comes in other materials too) that goes around the base of the shaft or under the balls and around the base of the whole package. It serves as a low-grade tourniquet of love. You put it on him before he's hard or completely hard. Beginners should use a stretchy cock ring or one with a buckle or Velcro so you can take it off when you want to. And don't leave it on for more than twenty minutes. Here's the scoop on two popular rings.

"I WANT A COCK RING THAT VIBRATES."

Try the Sonic Ring Kit. The nubs, spokes, and spikes encasing the ring add "ohs," and by tucking a small vibe, you can really take it up a notch.

What our customers say:

"My boyfriend and I had never used a cock ring before, but for $20, we figured even if this one didn't work, at least we hadn't wasted too much money on it. This one is great. The vibe is surprisingly powerful for something that size, and it worked like a charm. In short, my boyfriend went from hard, to rock hard, to steel hard. Incredible."

"I WANT A SUPER STRETCHY COCK RING."

The Elastomer Stretch Cock Ring stretches up to four times its size as you pull it over the penis and behind the testicles for the classic constriction that many men enjoy.

What our customers say:

"I bought this for my sweetie, and we thought it was going to break like the other mega-stretch ring, but it's really durable. It rocks."

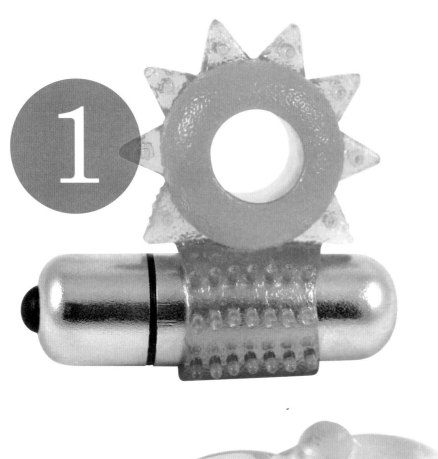

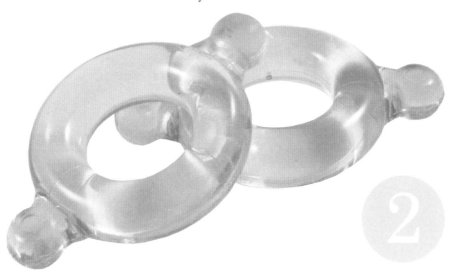

The BABELAND S·E·X Bill of Rights

Before we get into all of the wonderful ways to do it, we want to pause and share our babelicious credo, our ways to better lovemaking. It's all about permission. Permission to try new things, to take risks, to look foolish, to become a great big, heaving, yowling mess of desire and satisfaction. We'd like to create a new state of our own, a state of mind, Babeland … with hope that … (cue the fife music) one day every sexually active person will have the strength and guidance to get the most out of sex…(add marching drums) and the maturity to love themselves enough not to freak out when they encounter unexpected goo, a reluctant partner, or a wimpy orgasm. For we hereby declare that it's self-knowledge, self-expression, and overall joy that matter. We hold the following truths to be self-evident. Keep them in mind when you are naked with someone.

1

REMEMBER, YOU ARE SEXY— THE WHOLE OF YOU, INSIDE AND OUT.

Sex has a bigger zip code than the crotch zone. Use your entire body for good sex. Use your arms and knees and teeth. Stimulate your partner's scalp and thighs and earlobes. Incorporate all five senses into sex. It's better than theater in the round—both as performance and audience member. Growl, lick, listen, look around. And think. Your brain is the biggest sex organ you've got! Bring your head, your heart, your willingness and desire for connection. And use your lungs too. Breathe!

6

TAKE CHARGE OF SAFE SEX.

Since you have to live with the consequences, make safe sex and contraception happen. Don't wing it. If you want to use a condom, bring one and make sure to use it.

7

USE LUBRICATION.

Or at least have it nearby at all times. Wet and slippery feel good. Saliva and vaginal juices dry up quickly. Mouths and pussies have plenty to do already during sex—why not take the pressure off?

LOVE YOURSELF FIRST.

You deserve freedom from negative self-talk and internal criticism. If you are all worried about your hairy arms or your appendectomy scar, you're taking yourself out of the game. (We promise that your partner has got other things on their mind.) If you don't feel confident or worthy, you'll have a hard time being present, and you might even make some crappy, unsafe decisions. Remember, you are magnificent!

3

ENJOY THE JOURNEY.

Orgasms are great. We love them and wish you the best of them. However, the big O is not the whole point. A round of sex is over when you feel like it's over. The journey matters as much as the destination. You'll be missing the scenery if you are pumping away, gritting your teeth, and chanting, "I think I can."

4

OWN YOUR OWN ORGASM.

It's not your job to "make your partner come." And no one "gives" you an orgasm. Develop the skills and knowledge on your own to make yourself come (see Love Thyself, p. 40). Then bring that knowledge to the bedroom and share it with another person. If you're still precome orgasmic, just remember you have a lifetime to work it out, so keep the self-love flowing.

5

ASK FOR WHAT YOU WANT.

Have a system of communication. You don't have to sit down and plan a system of codes like a WWII submarine captain. But you gotta speak up. Good sex comes from giving updates and signals and receiving them. Check in with your partner using eye contact, sounds, and words. Dirty talk is fantastic for keeping momentum while checking in about satisfaction and consent. "I wanna fuck you from behind now. Would you like that?" Those are welcome words. We don't believe anyone has magical intuitive powers to be a good lover. It takes some effort.

LAUGH.

Sex at home isn't like the movies—neither the porn nor the big-screen kind. Your partner will kneel on your hair; parts will slip out of parts, you'll fart, the lubed-up butt plug will slip out and bounce across the floor. Be ready for things to go wrong and have a laugh about it. The bouncing butt plug will probably make you two laugh again when you think about it later. Don't take yourself too seriously and you'll have more fun.

9

DON'T BE AFRAID TO MAKE A MESS.

It's not often we get to rut around like animals. That's part of the treat. So try not to be too sensitive about goop flying about. By the time you are done there might be some spit, lady juices, semen, even pee and poop that make their way into your bed and onto your person. Just take a shower, no biggie.

10

KEEP GROWING.

Over a lifetime your desires change, and so does your body. So change up your sexual routine to fit what you need. Better yet, try not to have a sexual routine. Break patterns and try new things, just for the sake of newness and surprise. Variety is the spice of sex.

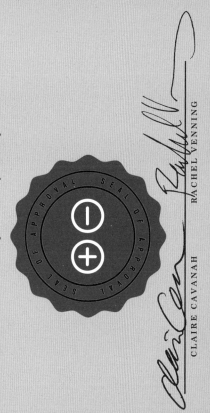

CLAIRE CAVANAH   RACHEL VENNING

CHAPTER 4

TURNING ON, TUNING IN:

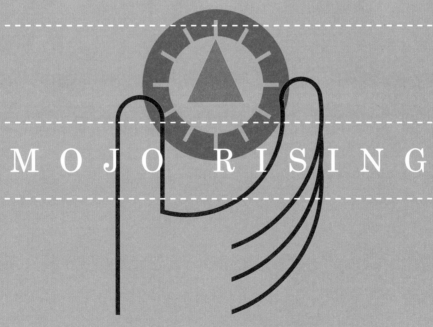

MOJO RISING

THE JOYS OF IGNIT

There's more to sex than sticking various parts into available holes. Obviously. There's kissing and **grinding** and undressing or dressing up in something **enticing**. There's teasing and talking and whispering. **Sharing fantasies.** So many wonderful,

NG YOUR ENGINE

exciting ways to build anticipation and enjoy the feeling of your **mojo rising**. In fact, sometimes feeling turned on can be satisfying all by itself, whether you're alone or with a partner. Parts going into holes ... that's an optional bonus.

KISS ME, KISS ME, KISS ME

Remember when kissing was all you did? Maybe in junior high or high school your technique wasn't the best, but the thrill was huge. Kissing is so intimate because all of your major sense receptors—eyes, ears, nose, and mouth—are hovering in close range, sensing up a little love storm. It's intense and personal. And it's common for couples who have lost that loving feeling to quit kissing—even though they're still having sex. We say that kissing merits your full attention and maybe even a refresher course. Yay, frenching!

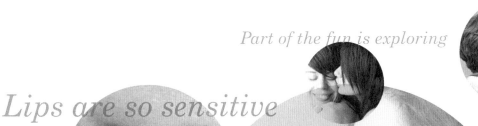

Part of the fun is exploring

Lips are so sensitive

Variety is nice

Invite your partner's tongue into your mouth

KISSING 101:
A REFRESHER COURSE

"Follow me."

Yes, there's a time and place for the grab-partner-and-mash-face move. But in general, it's super sexy—as well as polite—to start soft and ramp up from there. Brush your lips, slightly parted, against your partner's and see what happens. Lips are so sensitive that a delicate touch can send out (and bring in) a tidal wave of excitement. Let your tongue touch the lips and see what happens. If the kissee's lips part, then your tongue is invited in. But don't overstay your tongue welcome. Variety is nice. Try sucking on your partner's lower lip for a few seconds, even nibble a little. Invite your partner's tongue into your mouth by dipping yours in and pulling it back, as if to say, "Follow me." Part of the fun is exploring and seeing what your special friend responds to. And it's easier to read responses during kissing than, say, oral sex, because you're right near the eyes and your mouths are in contact and all the feedback is quite direct. But no need for mind reading either. Stop and talk. You can say, "OK, now I'm going to give you my idea of the perfect make-out kiss," then go to town. And after you've rendered your kissee helpless, say, "Now it's your turn!"

MORE MAKE-OUT TIPS

✓ **KISS BEYOND THE FACE.** Kiss the collarbones, earlobes, shoulders.

✓ **DON'T FORGET THE NECK.** Kiss the side of the neck, hollow of the neck, nape of the neck. The neck is an underserved area that's sensitive and holds lots of tension. Love it up.

✓ **USE YOUR TONGUE IN DIFFERENT WAYS.** Your tongue can be soft or hard, flat or pointy. (Use a hard and pointy tongue in small doses, lest you be mistaken for a lizard.)

✓ **KEEP YOUR HANDS BUSY BUT NOT FRANTIC.** Don't let your arms lie there like a lox. Touch your partner's face, cradle the head, bury your hands in your partner's hair, stroke a neglected inner thigh or two. Grab a handful of ass.

✓ **MAKE SOME NOISE.** No need for DVD commentary. But occasional "mmms" will make your mouth vibrate and give positive reinforcement.

✓ **FLOSS AS WELL AS BRUSH YOUR TEETH.** Brush your tongue too. This is more important (and more effective) than a good breath mint.

✓ **BREATHE.** Especially if you are nervous. Long, slow breaths through your nose will help ground you in the moment. Breathing through your nose will also keep you from drowning.

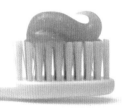

TOUCH ME,
TEASE ME

After the kissing starts, many couples lunge for each other's crotches. Just because **all the blood is rushing** there doesn't mean your hands have to. This is especially true for longtime couples. It's understandable to think, "Yeah, I know what comes next. Let's get to it." We've all done it. There's a time and place for a good quickie: the bathroom at a wedding, a freezing-cold camping trip, five minutes before your friends arrive for brunch, the back of a Chevy van in 1979. But when you hurry as a habit, you miss out. **Take time to caress and appreciate some other yummy parts: thighs, shoulders, tender toes.** Long-term couples can even designate a "Retro Night" when you grope around but don't fuck, like when you first hooked up. We promise it'll be hotter than acid-wash denim in a Wham! video.

MASSAGE THE SITUATION

Sometimes it's hard to transition from your frantic day, full of responsibilities and text messages and the squawking demands of others, into quiet, sexy times with your partner. So unplug. A massage can make this transition smoother and help you change gears. It's also a great way to savor all the many savory body parts. Make a special time and setting for a massage (or just for fooling around in peace). Turn off the gadgets, light some candles, turn on your mood-music playlist, bust out the yummy-smelling oils, and slather them on. You don't need training. Just do to your partner what you'd like to have done to your own back, butt, neck, and feet. Knead the muscles like tasty dough. Try to create a variety of sensations. Follow up with a light tickle from your fingertips. Next time? Your turn to receive.

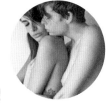

"F" IT! FROTTAGE!

While we're busy talking about massage and touching, there's the fine art of making yourself come by rubbing your tender parts on your sweetie's … anything. Some call it "dry humping," some call it "frottage" (from the French, who always keep it classy). There's the classic high school version in which two clothed people grind their pelvises together over clothes. It's hot, like a lap dance for two. The naked version feels nice. Women can (and do) rub their love buttons up against a lover's thigh, hard-on, hip bone, tailbone—anything firm and enticing. This is a good thing to do if your partner came first but you aren't quite there and you need a little something more to send you over the edge. It's fun for the rubbee to watch you ride 'em like a cowgirl. Yee-haw!

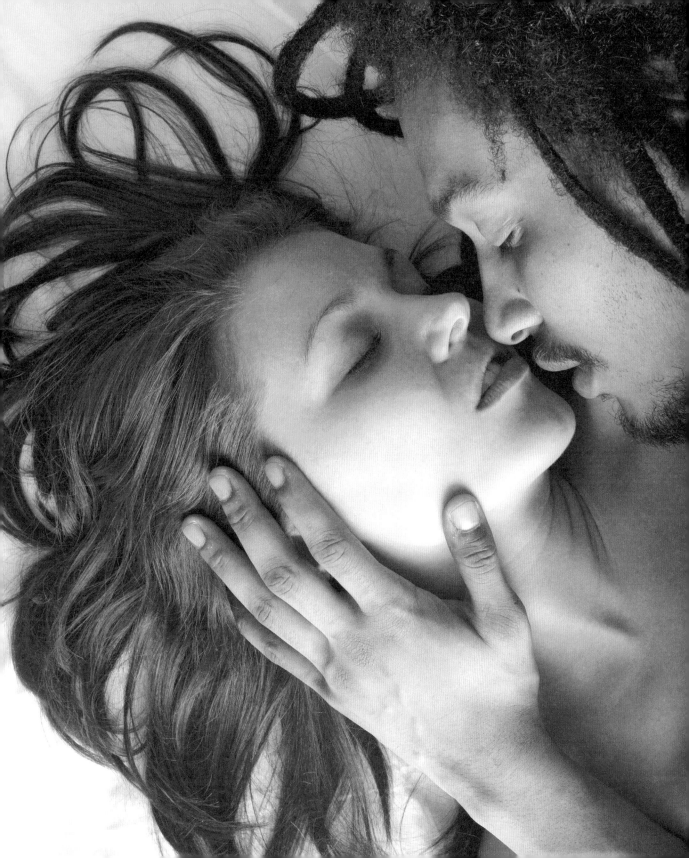

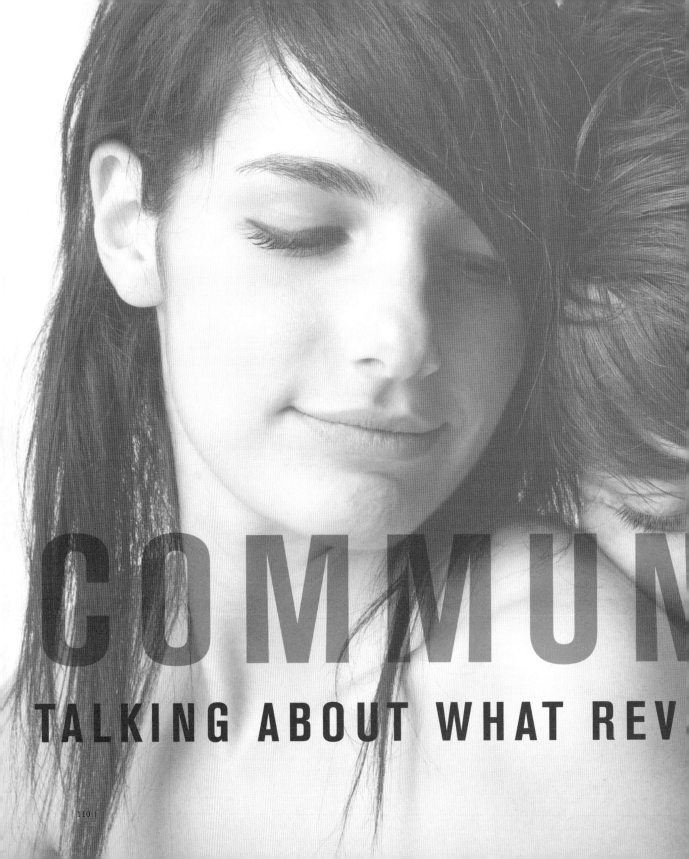

COMMUN
TALKING ABOUT WHAT REV

Whether you are trying to turn someone else on or you are helping someone to turn you on, at some point you have to talk. (Unless you are a really great mime.)

NO ONE IS A MAGICAL MIND READER

who can always intuit what to do when. Or how to touch what. If you don't talk, your sex life can become a frustrating guessing game, whether you are with a longtime partner or a new one. You run the risk of getting into a rut and doing the same routine over and over like some washed-up Vegas act. Talking about your desires, though not easy, opens doors. Really. It can lead you to new and exciting places, as well as a deeper sense of trust.

ICATION:

YOU UP

> "What do you think about when you make yourself come?"

> "Can you go a bit gentler on my clit? I'm a sensitive gal."

> "How about next time we try something a little bit different?"

> "I loved it when you went down on me, but maybe next time . . ."

CHATTING OUTSIDE THE BEDROOM

Most sex talk happens right before, during, or after sex play, and that's a good start. A postgame play-by-play can be a fun way to relive a great sexual experience and get feedback to make it even better next time. But there's an overview that can happen outside the bedroom—when your clothes are on and the blood is circulating not just in your pants but in your brain. We recommend putting aside time to talk sex with your partner somewhere more neutral than the bedroom (but still private, like on the patio with a cocktail). It's time to analyze the season, not just today's game. Take time to talk about how often you are getting naked together, how long you spend on different activities, things you want to try, what's working, and what you'd like to happen more frequently. The conversation can be scary and embarrassing, but no one is going to do it for you. And it's worth the risk of embarrassment to get more of what you want, and to give more of what your sweetheart wants. Try to be clear and positive.

FINDING THE WORDS

When in doubt, try saying, "I really liked it when you did _____," and go from there. As in, "I really liked it when you kissed my breasts for a seriously long time. That was unbelievably hot." Or "I really liked it when you went down on me, but … my clit got a little too much pressure and licking." Or "I love giving you head, but my neck gets tired and I'm worried you'll be annoyed if I stop." Then let the conversation flow from there. Maybe next time you go downtown, you

"Are you interested in a three-way?"

"I would love it if you paid more attention to my breasts."

"Do you like how I give you hand jobs?"

"I need more pressure on my clit."

"I really liked it when you . . ."

can stop and use your hand or a vibrator. Try to be an open-minded listener too. Prepare for some awkwardness. Prepare for funny moments and surprises, and more intimacy, too. Revealing more of yourself, and receiving kindness from your partner, leads to a closeness you may not expect. Be ready to learn a few of your sweetie's likes and dislikes… maybe your signature ball-licking move actually just tickles and frustrates him. Who knew? But now you do.

GO ON A SHOPPING SEXCURSION

Want another way to get a healthy conversation going outside the bedroom? We're not biased or anything, but a visit together—or alone—to a sex-toy shop will spark up your imagination. Especially if you aren't sure what you want. Just wander around and see what intrigues you. Maybe you never gave cock rings a moment's thought, but in person they look super sexy. Or maybe you can picture yourself at someone's tender mercy in supple restraints. Maybe the covers of the porno DVDs give you ideas. We welcome browsers at our store, especially if you're just trying to brainstorm. Or make a game of going on a shopping date and surprising each other with a $20 sex toy. Even if your partner buys something you don't like, it'll get you talking. Or giggling. And if your partner buys something you do like, it'll start more than a conversation. (If you don't have a store like Babeland nearby, you can browse online at babeland.com.)

THE YES/NO/MAYBE LIST

In many of our Babeland workshops, we hand out a "Yes/No/Maybe" list. It's a great tool for starting a chat. More like a game than homework. The rules are easy: Look at the list of sexual activities and put each one into a "Yes," "No," or "Maybe" column on a piece of paper. Just go with how you feel at the moment. There are no wrong answers, and you are not chiseling your choices in stone–you can change your mind later. When you're done, compare answers with your partner and see where you overlap. Instead of giving your loved one a hard time about their "Yes/No/Maybe" choices, try just asking, "Why no spanking?" (or whatever) and let it become a conversation. And remember that today's "No" could be tomorrow's "Maybe" and next month's "Yes."

SOME ACTIVITIES TO CONSIDER FOR YOUR "YES/NO/MAYBE" LIST:

- **Anal play**
  (with or without penetration)
- **Ball stretchers**
- **Blindfolds**
- **Bondage**
  (hands, feet, or both)
- **Caning**
- **Caressing**
- **Cock rings**
- **Cock sucking**
- **Consensual humiliation**
- **Cross-dressing**
- **Cuddling**
- **Cunnilingus**
- **Cybersex**
- **Dancing**
- **Dominance/submission**
- **Dripping hot wax**
- **Enemas**
- **Exhibitionism**
- **Fantasizing**

- **Finger-fucking**
- **Flogging**
- **Foot kissing**
- **Gags**
- **Gender play**
- **Golden showers**
- **Group sex**
- **Hair pulling**
- **Ice play**
- **Kissing**
- **Lap dancing**
- **Latex gloves/latex play**
- **Making videos**
- **Massage**
- **Multiple penetration**
- **Nibbling ears and neck**
- **Nipple clamps**
- **Oils and/or lotions**
- **Outdoor sex**
- **Paddling (leather, rubber)**
- **Paying for sex**

- **Phone sex**
- **Pinching**
- **Playing with sex toys**
  (vibrator, butt plug, dildo)
- **Public sex**
- **Reading erotica**
- **Rimming**
- **Role-playing**
- **Shaving**
- **Spanking**
- **Strap-on sex**
- **Stripping**
- **Sucking on nipples**
- **Talking dirty**
- **Threesome**
- **Tickling**
  (with hand, feathers)
- **Vaginal fisting**
- **Voyeurism**
- **Watching porn**
- **Writing a journal about sex**

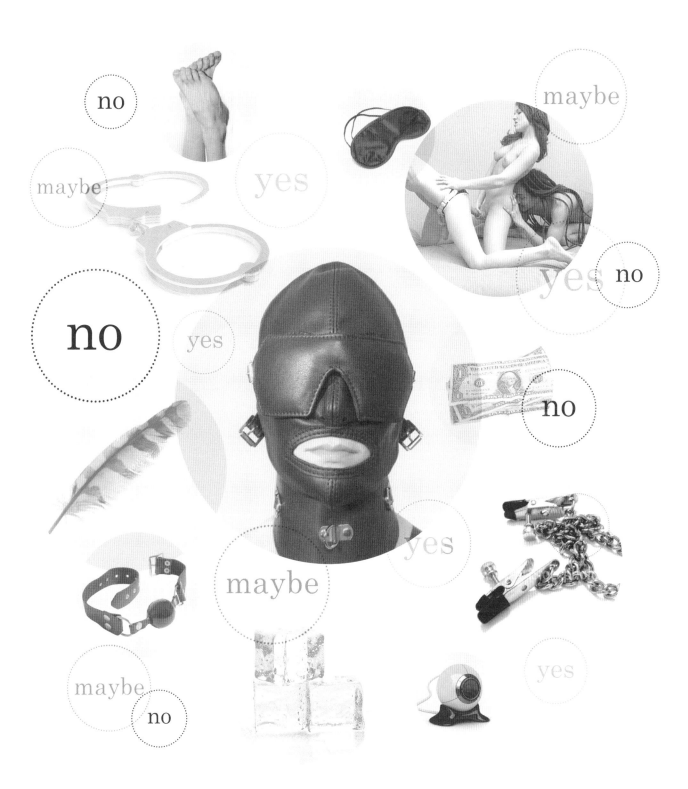

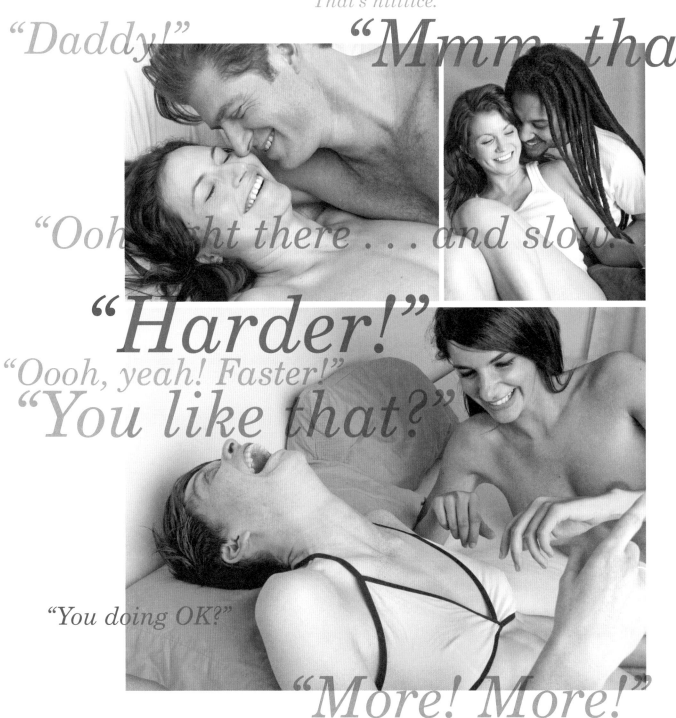

"That's niiiiice."

"Daddy!"   "Mmm... tha

"Ooh... ht there . . . and slow.

"Harder!"

"Oooh, yeah! Faster!"

"You like that?"

"You doing OK?"

"More! More!"

eels great!"

"Oh baby, that's it!"

CHATTING INSIDE THE BEDROOM

Once the action gets started in the bedroom (or on the couch, or on the kitchen counter, or in the back of that van), communication remains important. But keep it simple. You are working in a different gear. Focus more on the moment ("Mmm, that feels great") versus the bigger picture ("Why do you never initiate sex?"). The most important, basic tenet is to keep checking in with your partner—eye contact, body language, and sounds. Stay in touch. You're checking in for consent, and you're checking in for enjoyment. Consent doesn't have to sound like a permission slip from the school principal. A simple "You doing OK?" "You like that?" "Feel good?" will work fine. Really watch and listen for the answer and don't assume it's a yes. Be sensitive about correcting your partner. Instead of "Oh, don't do that!" try a more positive and specific, "That's nice, but go slow." Or one-worders like "Gentle," "Faster," "Harder," "Wait," and "There!" all work well. Words like "never" and "always" start fights. Be ready to receive the same kind of notes in return.

BEYOND WORDS

Be aware of good positive reinforcement–type sounds and moans versus silence. Notice body language. Someone pushing against you probably wants whatever you're doing to happen harder. Someone pulling back probably wants it lighter. Does an ass just scoot into your hands sometimes? Play with it.

TALKING DIRTY

Announcing what you want to do next is both sexy and a considerate way to make sure everyone's on board. It's also a good way to direct the action, as in, "I think it's time to spank you" or "Ooh, I need you inside me soon." Then there's dirty talk that's more about amping up the moment. "Mmm, you taste like honey." "Your cock is so rock hard." Some folks really enjoy letting dirty words fly during sex play, saying all the things they are not allowed to say with their clothes on: "I want to fuck your pussy!" "Suck my cock, Freaky Mama." It can be a totally fun form of cheerleading: "Oh, yeah, go! Do it! Do it!" Sometimes bedroom talk can slip into politically incorrect language: "Slut," "Daddy," "Bitch." Taboo words, like taboo behaviors, are exciting buttons to push, for better or worse. If certain words bother you or take you out of the moment, let your partner know: "Cunt is the only word I want you to use for my cunt," or "Cunt is the only word I do not want you to use for my puss." Some couples let the dirty talk flow. Others need to set the ground rules first. Or you can discuss it later. And of course, you are always welcome to stop what you're doing if it stops being fun.

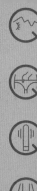

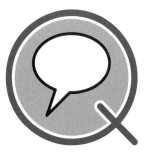

{ Q & A }

COMMUNICATION QUERIES

{Q} "Can you improve a bad kisser's kisses?"

{A} Well, bad kissing is totally subjective and a matter of chemistry and taste (as in desire, not taste buds, though they can come into play too). Some people like it hard, some people like it tender—one person's peck is another person's "Oh, puh-lease." What seems key to successful kissing is a game of lead-and-follow, with each partner taking a turn at initiating the tongue/lip action of the moment. The other person plays along and then has a turn at the lead. It's a lot like a good conversation, but with a very different unspoken vocabulary. If you are stuck with a "bad kisser," hopefully they will catch on to your lead and mirror back what you are doing. If one person is being too bossy and not giving up the lead, or being too passive and not following the lead, then you might have trouble. Again, it's like a conversation: both people have to give and take and pay attention. If you can't teach with your lips, you might have to speak up and have an actual chat—in which case, be very gentle and diplomatic. ("You are such a superfox, but I get a little overwhelmed when we kiss and need to come up for air more. Is that cool?")

"I have a hard time turning off my phone. My lover does too."

{Q}

{A} We all know that sex is a great stress reliever, but sometimes shutting down can be tough. Scheduling some sexy time can work, but more important, try to remind yourself how good and how connected you feel during and after sex. Putting techno-stuff on the shelf for the evening requires planning, willingness, and, for many, a reward system: "If you put your computer and phone away, I will make you come and bring you ice cream afterward." If doing it with your sweetie is less appealing than Facebook, a reluctance to have sex could be a sign of deeper problems. Are you using work to avoid the fact that you just don't want to have sex with your partner? Talk about what's holding you back. As awkward as it might be, it's still better than pretending that everything is OK.

"I move my boyfriend's hand to where I want it, and he doesn't like it."

{Q}

{A} Some people really like to be the choreographer, not just a dancer. You get points for trying to communicate, but he doesn't want to receive that message (at least not in that way at that time).

• Ask him about it. If he says he doesn't like having his hand moved for him, next time use your words instead. If he wants to run the show in the bedroom, give him some pointers when you're not in bed, then see if your sweetie works those notes into his horizontal naked dance with you. If he doesn't, he may need a more direct message from you.

• Could you be overcontrolling? Maybe once, try letting your partner be in charge with no help or hints from you. Maybe it'll be great. Hopefully your sweetheart will let you be the boss in return.

• If this is just one among many symptoms of bullheadedness, it's possible he can't be taught and it's time to move on to someone who's more considerate and flexible.

"I feel like a moron talking dirty, like I'm in a bad play."

{Q}

{A} Talking dirty does take a little nerve, like being onstage. But you've got an audience of one (unless you're in a three- or four-way, of course) who is probably very receptive to your performance. A really good starter script for dirty talk is simply this: say what you are going to do, then do it, then say you did it. Example: "I'm gonna suck your dick." (Dick sucking, stage left, with feeling.) Then, "I just sucked your dick!" It's hard to argue with that. Need a rehearsal? Practice by yourself in a mirror, just to get used to saying the words. Another easy warm-up: dirty texting. If iPhones and BlackBerries must invade our world, why not take advantage? Text a quick "I can't wait to eat you out." "I'm so wet thinking about tonight." "I love your cock." Be sure you have the right number before you hit "send."

MOVIE NIGHT

WATCHING PORN TOGETHER

At Babeland, we're big fans of porn, especially porn in which the women really look like they're getting off. We're also fans of porn that isn't so mainstream, in which the stars haven't had a lot of plastic surgery and real couples—gay or straight—with real chemistry burn up the screen. Of course, porn was basically invented to ignite your imagination, and there's something out there for everyone. It can certainly get two fires burning together. Make every other Tues-day into Skin Flick Night. Take turns going out and buying or renting a movie. There's also plenty of porn online. Watching a sexy movie with a lover can feel surprisingly intimate, maybe because it's something people usually do alone or clandestinely. You may find that once the movie gets going, you just start touching each other—almost like you are joining in the action on-screen. We are visual creatures, so take it all in and let your eyes enjoy.

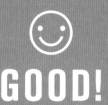

GOOD!

Reasons to enjoy porn...

Skilled performances!

The people in porn movies aren't always cast for their acting chops, but they can be amazing sex performers. Agile, creative, enthusiastic—they put on a lively show to tap into your lust.

Variety!

Think about it: zillions of porn movies have been made showing the same few physical acts (oral, vaginal, and anal sex). So their challenge is to show the same-old-same-old in a new way. Who knew that aliens doing it while riding in a donkey cart could be so hot?

Gives you ideas!

Porn stars try to present the sex act in new ways you can think about and even try. As in, "Honey, if we carpeted our stairs, could we do that too?" Porn helps you experiment.

Voyeurism!

It's a safe and legal way to see what you can't see anywhere else. What do other cocks and pussies look like? (Albeit sex stars' cocks and pussies, but still.) What does female ejaculation look like? How round and big can ass cheeks really be? Fascinating!

BAD!

Keep these factors in mind lest porn lead you astray...

Problem-free sex!

She doesn't yelp when he bumps his dick into her cervix too hard. Every position is apparently perfect ecstasy. Cell phones don't ring, and the super doesn't stop by to check the radiator valve (unless that's a plotline and he's hung like an elephant).

Smooth and perfectly fit bodies!

They may be easy on the eyes (if you enjoy super enhanced breasts) but can wreak havoc on the self-esteem. Think of porn actors as athletes who train all the time. You probably have a job and eat French fries every now and then.

Mega-erections!

Guys with cocks the size of telephone poles look like they can stay hard through a screening of the entire *Lord of the Rings* trilogy. Keep in mind these fellows are probably taking Viagra and jerking off, or even just taking breaks between scenes. And funny how they always come right when they want to. They don't call it a "money shot" for nothing.

Rushing in the back door!

Anal sex in porn can be a bad example to follow. Directors don't want to spend the screen time coaxing the butt hole to the relaxed and happy place it requires. They either do the coaxing beforehand—by prepping the rectum with a butt plug—or they don't do it at all and ram on in with lots of lube. Do not try that at home.

Faked orgasms!

We hope there are some real ones in there. But remember, these are performers. Since we can see evidence when a guy comes, apparently we have to hear it from the ladies. Maybe they get paid by the decibel.

It's not a study guide!

Porn is not a good substitute for sexual knowledge, so enjoy it, but don't use it as a how-to manual.

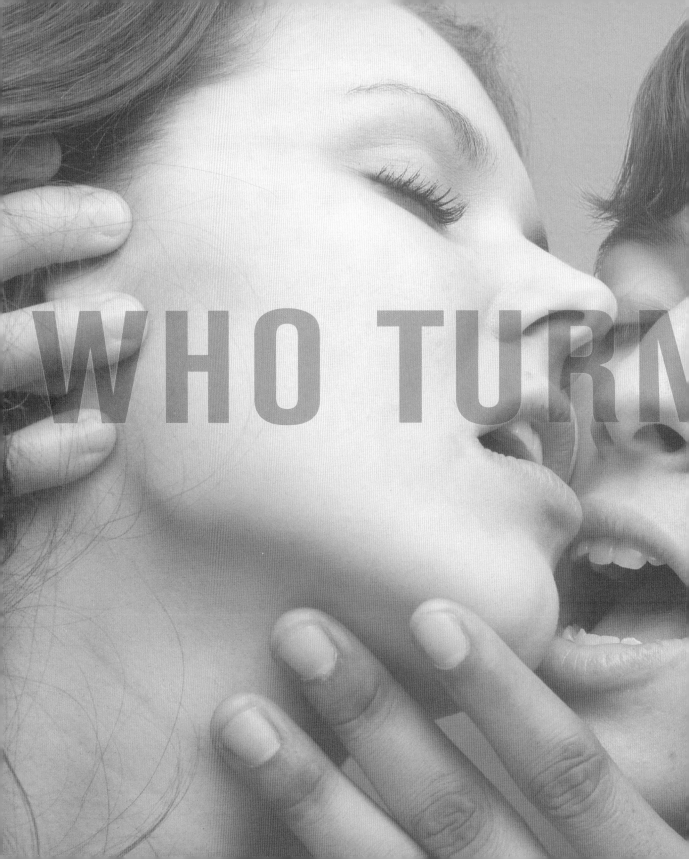

S YOU ON?

Notice whom you are drawn to and whom you can imagine fondling and fucking while walking down the street. It's a fun exercise in fantasy. Notice also if you are drawn to extremes of manliness or girlishness—or do you dig androgyny? Keeping a running checklist in your head of qualities you definitely need in a lover ("I like tall, skinny poet-type guys with tattoos") can be limiting. Then what about the beefy lifeguard dude or the butchy barista at your café? Maybe they are your soul mates—or really good kissers for a one-night make-out stand.

YOU ONLY LIVE ONCE, SO WHY NOT EXPERIMENT?

Try someone outside the range of your usual type—perhaps just with a different dress style, height, or body shape. And keep checking in with yourself, because desires change over a lifetime.

Labels are for clothes.

A.B.E. ALWAYS BE EXPLORING

You may only have sex with people of one gender for your whole life. On the other hand, it's fun to get out and explore a bit. You may feel that the label "straight" or "gay" really fits you. But even strongly identified lesbians have been known to fuck the occasional man, and if it weren't for straight men who have sex with men, highway rest stops would be a lot less crowded. Plenty of mostly straight women enjoy a threesome with another woman here and there. And there are plenty of people who confidently identify as "bi." Let your orientation be a source of pride, not a container that keeps you... contained.

I.D. PLEASE: GENDER IDENTITY

Gender identity is something we all absorb and live out, from the moment a baby girl is dressed in pink or a little boy hears, "No, you may not wear Mommy's necklace." Whether we think about it or not, there are messages all around us. Look at the images of masculinity and femininity on TV, in advertising, or at family gatherings. These messages affect what we wear, how we walk, whom we date, and much more. The strict rules can be limiting. Even though *American Idol* has sanctioned "guy-liner" makeup, we've got a ways to go. We still have to choose between the men's and women's public bathrooms at the airport, each with its own distinct icon on the door. In real life, there is a broad spectrum of gender—from cowboy supermacho dude-

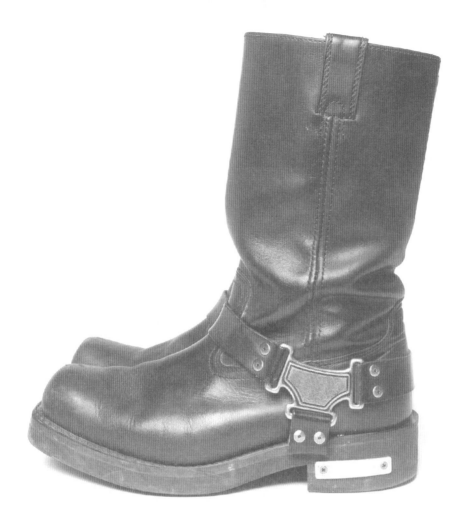

ness on one end, to young David Bowie androgyny in the middle, to Glinda the Good Witch feminine on the other end. We all fall somewhere on that continuum. We can think about what masculine and feminine mean to us—what we want to be, and what we crave. What persona feels good and comfortable and sexy? It's fine to move around on the scale from year to year or day to day. Switch from your Timberlands to your Jimmy Choos and you just got girlier for the night.

GENDER OPTIONS: BODY VS. SOUL

For some people, the gender identity they choose to express does not match what's in their pants. The gender assigned at birth doesn't always feel right later. So there are choices. You can be assigned female at birth but dress in a masculine way. You can have a cock but dress and live as a woman. You can go a step further and start changing your body with hormones, which may help you feel more manly or womanly on the inside and change your outward appearance and sometimes your personality. Some people assigned male who identify as women get breast implants but keep their penises, which still provide pleasure. Female-assigned folks who identify as male may get surgery to remove their breasts but keep the vulva. "Transgender" doesn't mean resculpting your genitals—it means expressing a different gender than what you started with, by any means you choose.

DRESSING UP

Gender roles, of course, are a huge part of mating and dating and turning on. Even animals wear special stripes and plumage when it's time to get it on. Clothes and makeup—which you can put on and take off at will—are fun to play with. Clothes help you express gender, take it to an extreme, or try on a different one. Think of the zingy energy of a spiky high heel, a leather jacket, a push-up bra, biker boots. Don't you notice those when you are on the prowl? Do you have a go-to getup you wear when you want to seduce someone? Think of the power of a man's power suit. Now picture it on a woman. Sexy in a new way, right? Then there are wardrobe secrets for under your clothes—lingerie, garter belts, strap-ons. A guy can wear a cock ring under his innocent-seeming khakis. Tell your partner what you've got going on underneath, and in no time you'll be home having your wrapping ripped off. Or girls, make a wardrobe change into a harness and dildo. There's an excellent chance your partner—guy or girl—will be curious and excited about your strap-on. Use clothes to play and have fun. We are visual creatures, so give the eyes some treats. See how it feels.

Use clothes to play and **HAVE FUN.**

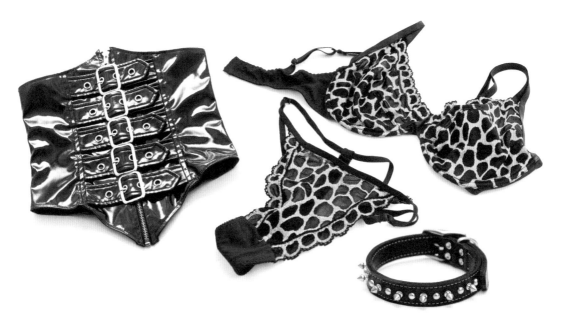

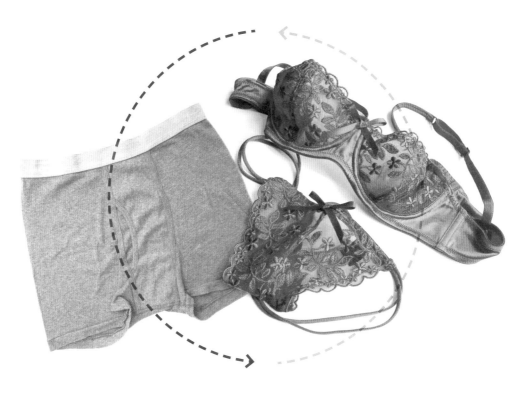

{ Try This at Home }

DRESSING GAMES

Switcheroo If you are a man/woman couple, dress each other in clothes of the opposite sex. You get to style your partner. If you are a man/man or woman/woman duo, try dressing up as a man and a woman–taking turns at who gets to wear the pants. Stay at home or take your new look out and about. Try having sex with your outfits still (mostly) on. Or no matter what your pairing, try all three: man/woman, woman/woman, man/man. Have fun!

Undertow Wear underwear of the opposite sex under your clothes for a day. See what kind of energy that gives you as you sit through a boring budget meeting.

Sugar daddy/mama Shop for a dream item you want your sweetheart to wear– a see-through shirt, tight jeans, stripper heels, whatever flies your kite.

FANTASY ROLE-PLAYING

Go to a Halloween party and you'll see women dressed as nurses, cheerleaders, flight attendants, plus the occasional sexy bumblebee. Guys will dress as pirates, athletes, vampires. These are all sexually charged fantasies (we do not judge if bumblebees are your thing). There's tons of gender play too—notice the guys dressed as cheerleaders, the girly chick who's now Elvis. Why limit that kind of fun to one night a year? Especially if you and your partner can work together and dress up for a little sex play. Of course, you don't need costumes for role-play (though they can be a hoot—French maid, anyone?). You just need a character and some motivation, and you can make up the script. There are some classic role-playing scenarios: doctor and patient, boss and secretary, teacher and student, prisoner and guard, queen and servant. As you can see, these games are often about power relationships where someone is

in charge and the other has to do their bidding. But not always. It can just be a new point of view that you want to try on: stripper and client, rock star and groupie, high school football player and, yes, cheerleader (or how about two football players?), two strangers on the subway who decide to do it, astronaut washed up on a desert island after five years in space and an islander. Just agree to the scenario and seduce each other in character. You may giggle a bunch, but that's part of the fun. Really tongue-tied? Act out a scene from a movie you find sexy.

EXPLORING OTHER FANTASIES

Then there are the many fantasies in which you get to play yourself. What do you think about when you masturbate? Can you tell your partner so he or she can make it come true? ("You wash me head-to-toe in a bubble bath, getting in all the cracks and nooks of my body. You wash my hair, comb my hair, then lay me down and fuck me slowly while I keep my eyes closed.") You can talk through a fantasy, telling a story while your partner masturbates—sort of like in-person phone sex. ("We are in a museum in Paris filled with armor and paintings and porcelain dishes. I start touching your cock through your pants until I feel you are hard. When no one is looking, I grab you, and we duck behind a tapestry, where I unzip you and start sucking.") Bonus: you can also do this by phone when you are apart.

OPENING UP THE BOUNDARIES

Maybe the idea of being stuck with one person sounds boring. There are lots of ways to expand the playing field and bring fantasy into real life. You can invite someone you both find attractive to have sex with you. Or another couple. Maybe pairing up isn't who you are. Lots of folks live poly (short for polyamorous) lifestyles. Some have multiple serious relationships going at once. Some have one primary partner and other relationships of lesser importance (but that are still significant). Some people like to go to sex clubs and swingers' conventions for quick, commitment-free hookups. There are lots of ways to structure your romantic life, so skip the white-picket-fence lifestyle if it ain't you.

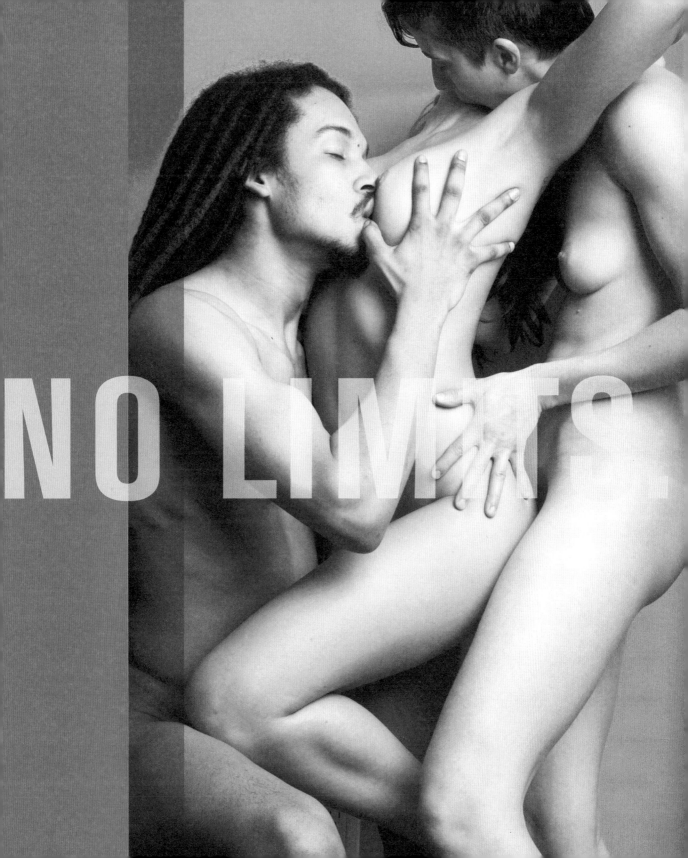

NO LIMITS

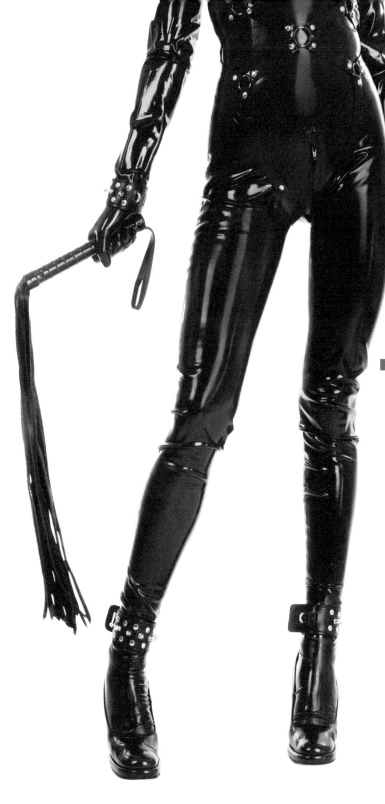

TIE ME

BONDAGE AND DOMINATION

Bondage can be a natural extension of role-playing games—the prison guard who cuffs his prisoner, the queen who ties up her servant for a spanking. It can also be fun on its own, with one person taking control and the other person submitting. For the bound person, there's a certain freedom in giving up all the power. You don't have to decide anything, you don't have to plan anything, and you don't have any responsibilities from being in charge all day. It's no accident that a dominatrix we know ties up a lot of overworked, stressed-out corporate CEOs—for them it's a relief. For the person tying the ropes, there's the excitement of seeing your partner all laid out and pretty—like a butterfly pinned to a cork board. And there's the thrill of being in charge, of having all the power. Your partner's body becomes your

BLIND MAN'S BLUFF

With permission, bind your partner—just hands, or hands plus feet. Add a blindfold and maybe even music so that the main sense you control is touch. Then pleasure your partner with oral sex. Bring them to the edge and then back away. When satisfied and in blisstopia, the bound person can be set free.

UP, TIE ME DOWN

personal playground, an instrument to make music on. And of course, trust is a big part. With bondage play, be safe, ensure the consent of both parties, be extra clear and communicative about what you are going to do, and agree on a "safe word" that stops the action quickly. Be sure you've agreed on the rules. (See below.) The main rule: when the bound person wants out, that's fine. No questions asked. Bondage won't work if just one of you is into it. Then it's kidnapping.

BONDAGE AND PLEASURE/PAIN SAFETY TIPS

• Before you play, agree on the menu of activities that you want to try. Stick to the menu.
• Never let someone you don't trust tie you up.
• Never tie up necks.

• Make sure bonds are not too tight and there's no pressure on joints like wrists and ankles. There should be a finger's width of space between skin and restraints.
• Make sure the unbound person can free up the bound person easily and quickly.
• Keep safety scissors nearby in case of emergency.
• Don't tie a standing person's ankles together, and don't tie someone to a chair that could tip over.
• When starting out, just do this for twenty minutes or so to see how your body and anxiety levels fare.
• If you are bound and start to feel tingling (bad tingling in your hands, for example), tell your partner to undo the bind.
• Agree to code words like "yellow" for "OK, but back down, less of this" and "red" for "Let's be done with this altogether."

PLEASURE & PAIN

SM PLAY

Many who love bondage also love to explore the edges and overlap of pleasure and pain. Combining the whole shebang is BDSM (bondage, domination, sadomasochism). You can enjoy SM play with bondage or à la carte. "But I hate pain. Why would I want it on purpose?" you might ask. In SM play, the pain is different from a toothache or stubbing your toe (both of which suck). The pain in SM doesn't hurt like that.

IT'S AN INTENSE SENSATION THAT BLOSSOMS INTO PLEASURE.

The thrill of taking the pain "for" the other person can also be a big turn-on. It's about finding your boundaries and pushing them further. It's about building up sexual tension even more for a megawatt release.

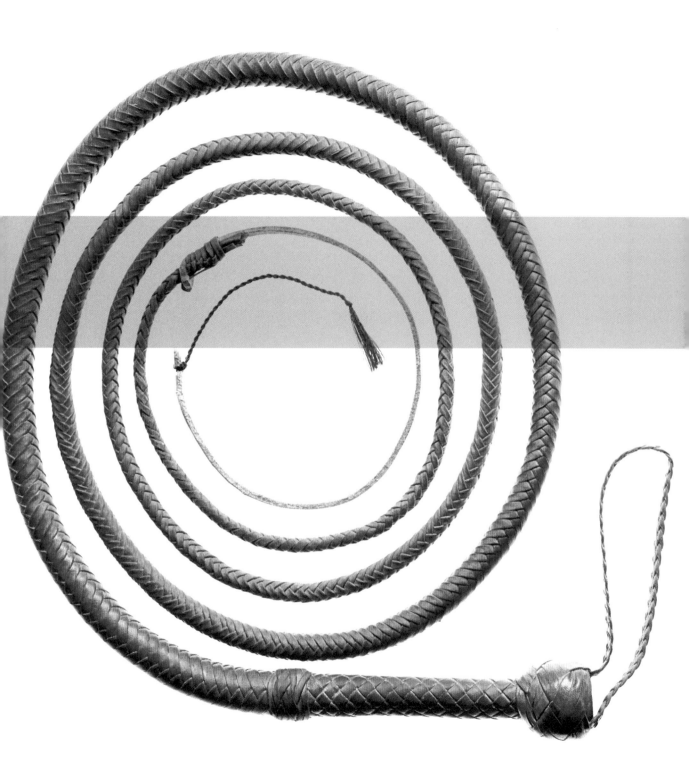

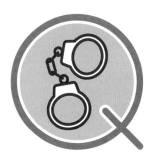

FANTASY/ BDSM

{Q} ## "How do I even begin trying SM play?"

{A} Start by talking to your partner when you're not in bed. BDSM play requires partners to be equally game with somewhat matching curiosities and desires. It doesn't work if just one of you is into it. Where to start? Have a chat and discuss the things you want to try. The "Yes/No/Maybe" list (p. 114) can be helpful here. Maybe pick one activity for your first time—say, spanking. (Spanking is a good, classic starter for pleasure/pain exploration.) You want BD with your SM? Agree on that. With or without BD, SM play still involves one person giving and controlling the sensations and one person receiving them. Despite the outward appearance of a one-way show, really good SM is a dynamic exchange of power, in which each partner contributes equally to keeping the energy hot. If you are the sensation giver, get your partner aroused—kissing, grinding, giving orders. Take your time. When your partner is definitely turned on, add some spanks. The butt has nice padding, and a good spank sends shockwaves to the entire genital area. Striking the butt down lower, toward where it meets the thighs, feels better than spanking up high, by the tailbone. Add or subtract whacks depending on the response you get. Build up a rhythm. Add oral sex or penetration if you want. Pay close attention and don't assume your partner is OK. Check in with your eyes and with your words. Then let the sparks fly.

{Q} "What if I was into something with my partner one night but now I'm not into it anymore?"

{A} You have crossed a certain line of sexual behavior, and your partner assumes you are willing to stay there. But of course you can change your mind and take a break from such shenanigans. Or maybe you just wanted to cross this act off your bucket list and now you are done. That's fine. Consent is something that needs to be renewed and not assumed. Time to speak up outside the bedroom. Say something like, "Honey, that night of paddling/anal beads/nipple clamps/whatever was fun and hot. But now it's not getting my juices flowing. Can we take a break from that and do other stuff?" Of course that's a rhetorical question, and the answer is yes.

{Q} "I'm really into it and I want more—what's next?"

{A} The world of the SM community is nearly endless. There are play parties, conventions, campouts in the woods, leather contests, online groups (and we have workshops at Babeland!). Some folks who get into SM also have multiple relationships to express different sides of themselves. And there is a world of gear! Different kinds of ropes and restraints, paddles, canes, floggers, multitudes of whips, esoteric medical devices. Try popping "Folsom Street Fair" (a huge SM street fair in San Francisco) into your search engine and follow the links. You're off to the races.

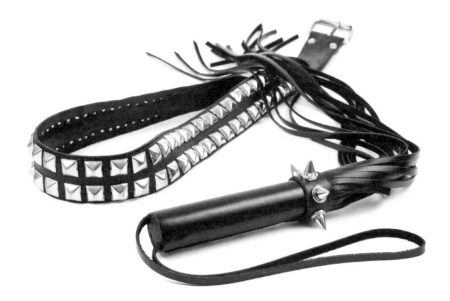

{THE BONDAGE GUIDE}

Soft as a feather or hard as a whip, the range of sensations people like to dole out and receive during sex varies wildly. In the erotic bubble of a scene, things that might normally be uncomfortable or hurt either aren't painful at all or hurt in a good way. Often with harder-to-take sensations, the receiver's body becomes flooded with endorphins that help transform sensations into something thrilling. Here are some toys to get you started:

"RESTRAINTS SEEM COMPLICATED. GOT ANYTHING SIMPLE?"

No need to install complicated hardware or perfect your Boy Scout knots to have someone pinned and completely at your mercy. The Under the Bed Restraint system is simple and discreet, and it sets up in a snap.

What our customers say:

"My boyfriend and I wanted an effective restraint system for some fun tied-down/control play. The kit was very easy and simple to install—and easy to hide under the bed! The straps are sufficiently sturdy and stay adjusted and the cuffs are incredibly soft and comfortable."

"I WANT NIPPLE CLAMPS THAT CAN BE LIGHT ON MY PARTNER BUT MORE INTENSE ON ME."

The very popular Tweezer Clamps easily adjust from light to tight. The rubber tips slip off for cleaning but stick for nipple clamping. A must-have for your toy bag!

What our customers say:

"This was my first venture into nipple clamps and these have been great. He and I both enjoy them. I especially like the heavy feel of the chain on my belly or in my hand, depending on who is wearing the clamps."

"WE'RE SORT OF A LEATHER COUPLE . . ."

Get a lover or playmate into the Panther Cuffs, and who knows how long they'll want to stay put! Soft black leather decorated with silver studs creates a classic look; the cuffs also sport a wide inner lining of soft leather for comfort and a thicker outer strap for sturdiness.

What our customers say:

"The leather the Panther Cuffs are made with is so soft and they aren't bulky like some other cuffs. I love that they are designed so that you can put a little padlock through the hole on the buckle to lock them on."

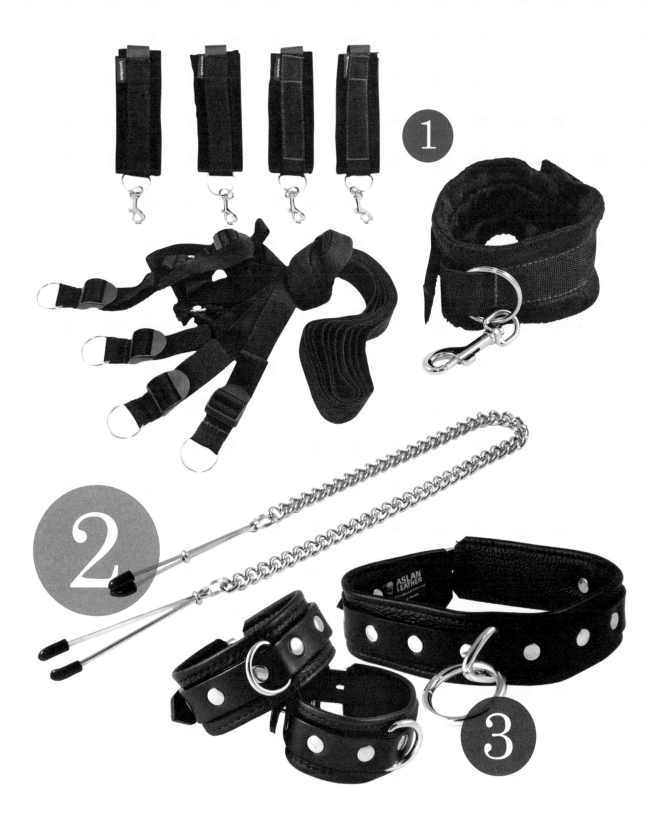

CHAPTER 5

GETTING OFF:

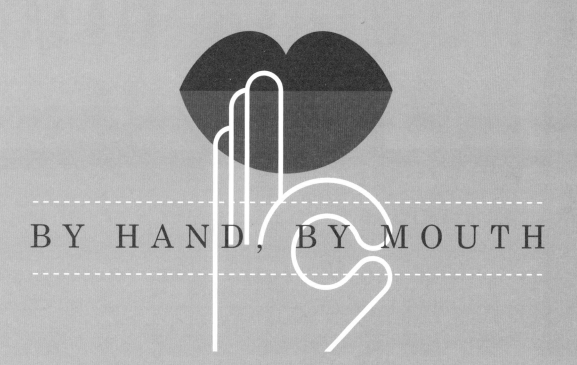

BY HAND, BY MOUTH

HAND JOBS, BLOW
and EATING PUSSY

GIVING AND RECEIVING ARE TWO OF LIFE'S GREAT TREATS.

These acts are designed purely to give pleasure—they put the "joy" in sexual enjoyment. Being able to give great sex in a way that's also fun for you is empowering. And chances are a little sex karma will kick in, and you'll receive some pleasuring back. Whether you are a novice or a dirty old dog,

WE BET WE CAN TEACH YOU SOME NEW TRICKS.

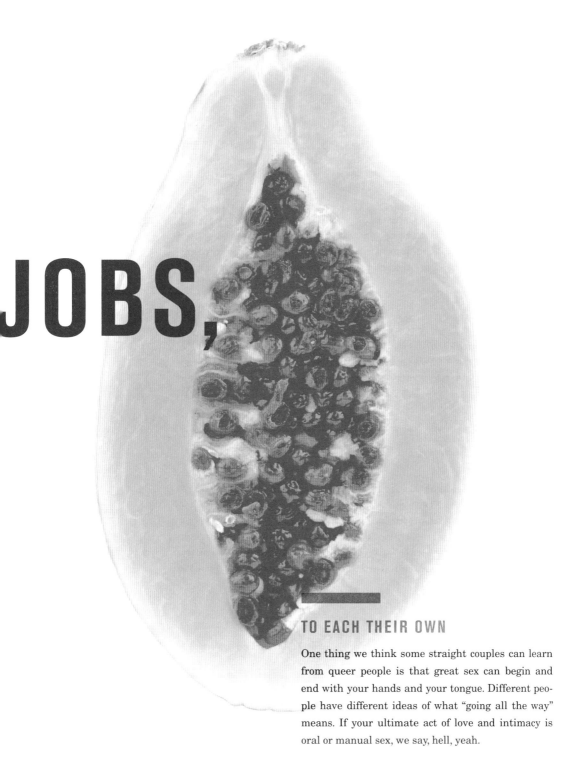

JOBS,

TO EACH THEIR OWN

One thing we think some straight couples can learn from queer people is that great sex can begin and end with your hands and your tongue. Different people have different ideas of what "going all the way" means. If your ultimate act of love and intimacy is oral or manual sex, we say, hell, yeah.

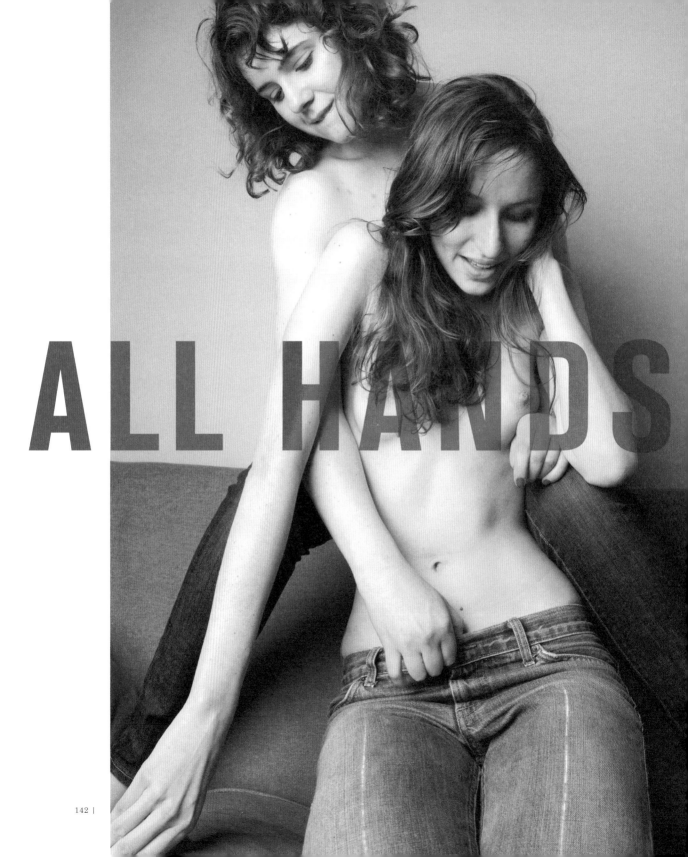

ALL HANDS

Why we love using our hands:

1 **Fingers are more dexterous than dicks or dildos.**

2 **You can enjoy full-body contact while using them.**

ON CLIT

3 **You can penetrate with anything from the pinkie to the whole mitt.**

4 **You and your partner can perform simultaneously.**

5 **Hands are lower maintenance than toys. No batteries!**

MANUAL LABOR OF LOVE: HAND JOB ON A WOMAN

Hands can actually do so much more than dicks and dildos. Did you ever see a penis play the cello? Or a dildo crochet a doily? Thought not. The dexterity and versatility of fingers are amazing. The hand can use fingers together or apart. It can make big or small movements. Hands can be stiff or flexible. Hands can massage. Hands can open a bottle of lube and squeeze. There are many good-time ways the hand can please the pussy.

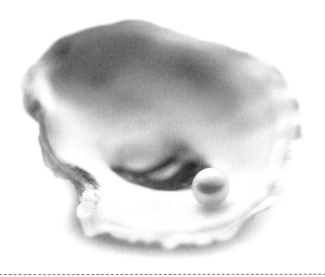

FUCK A WOMAN WITH YOUR HAND

For the basics, check out the section where we talk about ways a woman can jill off with her hand (p. 56). And, heck, if you're a gal, you probably already have some idea of

HOW TO EFFECTIVELY POLISH THE PEARL.

But every body is different. Here's the rub (har har): if you are working your hand magic on a woman, we want you to give up the goal of bringing her to orgasm. Let it go. If it happens, hurray, but it's not the be-all and end-all. When petting pussy—someone else's pussy—it's all about exploring, listening, and feeling for feedback to get her to a happy place, with or without explosion.

PREP SCHOOL

Clip your nails! Long nails, jagged nails, and nails with sharp corners all turn into lethal weapons when nearing a clit or vagina. Have water- or silicone-based lube nearby so there's less pressure on her juices to do all the slip-sliding. Grab any vibes or toys she wants.

IN POSITION

It's nice to lie on your side, right next to the lucky lady. Make sure your dominant hand is available. Approach her from above so your hands can touch her from the same angle hers do—the kind of touch she is used to. Resting your wrist on her mons is a good home base for finger exploration. Or try reaching around from behind her while spooning. Or do it standing up in the stacks of the library.

GETTING STARTED

As in all good sex play, there's no need to pounce on the genitals. Make out for a while. Tickle her thighs. Circle her nipples. Run your fingers through her pubic hair (if she has any). Maybe caress and massage the outer labia before diving in.

WATCH, FEEL, LISTEN, AND LEARN

Once her motor is running, pay attention to feedback, ask questions, and even ask her to show you how she touches herself. What kind of rhythms does she create? See if you can take over. Let her fingers rest over yours and guide you. Once you get the hang of it, go it on your own. You don't have to stick to her rules, but watch and listen for her response. When in doubt, start anything gently and slowly, then increase pressure and speed. Build up a rhythm.

CHECK YOUR INDICATORS

A woman is a little tougher to read than a dashboard, but so much more interesting. Moans and pushing into you are good signs. You can lose some of the guesswork by asking questions. In a sexy voice say, "Does this feel good?" "Does your cunt like that?" We are big fans of using dirty talk to actually communicate. And can you see or feel the physical signs of her getting excited? Her labia and clit are probably getting engorged, the skin is getting darker and more flushed, and the juices are getting juicier. If no warning lights come on, then keep driving.

A NOTE ON THE LOVE BUTTON

The center of her V-universe is the clitoris. Make sure it's happy, but don't jump all over it unless you get a pretty serious written invitation—with calligraphy and stuff. The clit is sensitive, so approach with awareness. There are a lot of ways to please it indirectly: touching it through the hood, playing with the inner labia, circling around it. Pretend it's a peeled grape covered in nerves. Because it basically is.

STOP AND SMELL THE ROSES

Show your sweetheart how into her you are by stopping to smell or taste the fingers you're using. If she's at all self-conscious about her scent, this will set her at ease. And if she's not, it's another way to communicate your desire to go down on her in the near future.

GET IN THERE!

She'll let you know when she wants fingers inside. Go in one joint deep and circle, then try two joints, and maybe all the way in. Keep an eye on her responses and take it from there. It's up to you to decide how to play it, slowly building up the intensity or fucking her madly. As she opens up, add more fingers. You'll be happy if you have lube on hand. Most of the sensation of fucking is from the sliding in and out and the impact. If she isn't letting you know to keep it right where it's at or to back off, go for it. Why do lesbians love girls in muscle shirts? Because when we get a nice look at those built shoulders and defined biceps, we know we can count on a good, solid fuck.

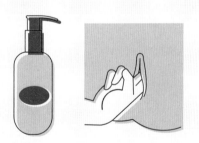

The tenets of successful finger fucking: have lube, go in slowly, and add more fingers as she opens up.

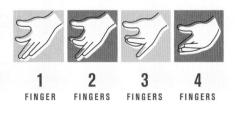

1	2	3	4
FINGER	FINGERS	FINGERS	FINGERS

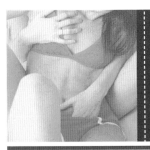

FANCY HAND MOVES FOR HER

The Octopus

Hands and legs are wrapping around her while you polish her pearl. Feels like a nice big bear hug combined with an equally lovely hand job.

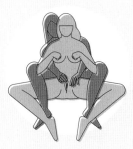

Three's Company

Take three fingers. Use the first and third to spread the outer labia and the second to run up and down the inner labia.

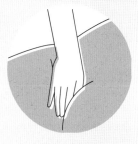

Palm Sunday

This is good if she loves to masturbate with indirect external pressure (a.k.a. humping things). Place your whole palm over her mons and massage in small, steady circles. Make sure there is contact and pressure just above the clit.

The Bend Over

She's on her hands and knees while you reach through from behind. A perfect opportunity for tickling her ass to boot.

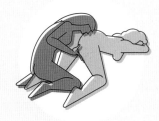

Circling the Perimeter

Gently tickle in circles that trace around the edge of the vaginal opening. Reverse direction and circle some more. Go in a little deeper if she's liking it.

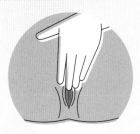

The Light Switch

Use your first two fingers or just your middle finger to lightly slide up and down her vag like you are flipping a light switch. Start by going up and down the labia and just inside the vaginal opening. You can try it lightly on her clit too.

G-WHIZ

G-SPOTTING WITH FINGERS

If you find a steady rhythm and your partner is really turned on, it could be time to do a little G-spot spelunking. With your hand palm-up, slide two fingers about two inches in and feel the ceiling of the vagina for a rougher patch of skin with sort of a bulge under it. That's the G-spot (and the bulge is the urethral sponge, a.k.a. the female prostate—see p. 20). Massage the G-spot with the "come here" gesture of the fingers. Stroke, don't poke. More vigorous fucking works for many women. Some women can take it for a long time, and multiple orgasms are common, so givers, engage your core, keep breathing, and know that maybe you will skip the gym tomorrow. If she suddenly feels like she's going to pee, that could mean that she's going to ejaculate (releasing a harmless liquid that is NOT pee). Encourage her to let it rip, and if you are having a lucky day, she might even orgasm and shoot all over you.

Amazing what only two fingers can accomplish.

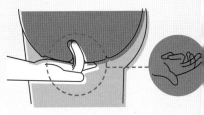

FISTING IS NOT JUST A POLITICAL GESTURE

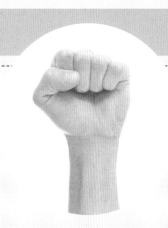

As handiwork on a gal heats up, she might yearn for more fingers to fill her up, especially if her vagina is expanding and opening on the inside from excitement. Once you get to three fingers (or even four), the shape of your hand stops you from going more than finger-distance inside. You may want to try fisting, which does not involve anything as rough as the name implies. Vaginal fisting is putting an entire hand–with great care, love, patience ... and lube–into your sweetie. It's an act of trust and incredible intimacy that's exciting and humbling and thrilling all at once. It's not for everyone, but if you love getting finger-fucked, you enjoy the feeling of being filled up, and you totally trust your partner, then fisting might be for you.

HOW TO GO TOTALLY DIGITAL

1 Donning a latex glove for fisting will help your hand glide inside. Plus, latex gloves equal safer sex.

2 A good position for her is lying on her back with knees bent and legs relaxed. Using liberal amounts of lube, insert one finger at a time until there are four inside. If your palm is up toward the sky, it will be more comfortable for her and keep the knuckles from bumping her pubic bone.

3 She can help by coordinating her breathing, exhaling as fingers go in. Go slow. Tease. After you have four fingers inserted, withdraw them and add a thumb to the mix, putting all five fingertips together to make the shape of a bird's head. The idea is to make the narrowest shape possible. With patience, lube, and maybe a little twisting motion of the "swan's beak," your whole hand can slide past the muscular ring around the vaginal opening.

4 Once inside, your hand will naturally fold up around the thumb into, yes, a fist–surrounded by warm vaginal walls. Your hand can rock a little, slowly twist, or clench and unclench a bit. Whatever feels good. It's the intense opening and the closeness that feels amazing and transcendent for so many folks.

5 To undo, exit with the care used to get in. (If there is a feeling of suction, break the seal by slipping a finger from the free hand into the vaginal opening.) She can bear down on her vaginal muscles as you slowly pull out, unfolding your hand along the way. She will feel the effects on her inner V-muscles for a few days and maybe even spot a little blood. She may also feel she's added a thrilling new aspect to her sex life!

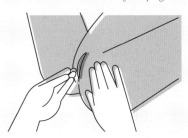

Make a bird's head with your fingers.

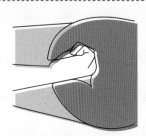

Once inside, your hand will naturally fold into a fist.

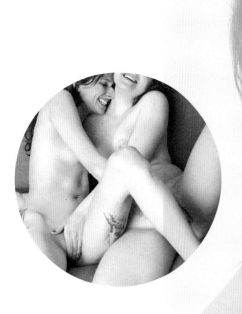

MUTUAL MASTURBATION

Try reaching across and hand-servicing each other at the same time. This is nice when sitting side-by-side on a couch or in a car (high school flashback, anyone?), or lying next to each other in bed. The huge advantage is that you can see each other and even kiss. You can also do it lying head-to-feet, feet-to-head—then you get a front-row view of your partner's nether parts. And all these are very safe forms of sex.

TWO-WAY LIVE SEX SHOW

Oh, the joy of hand-jobbing yourself while your partner watches and does it too. It's like your own live porn! You get to be voyeur and exhibitionist at the same time. Some ideas and variations: take turns instead of going at the same time. Or try to sync it so you come together. This can be difficult—have fun and don't make yourselves crazy. Add toys!

TOYS! ANAL!

If your hand gets tired, you can let a vibrator do some of the work. (See p. 68 for ideas on vibrator play.) If she is excited, you can bring pleasure from the plethora of nerves around the butt hole, which is right there anyway. Use the other hand so that the fingers don't go from butt hole back to vulva and cause an infection. Try lube while circling around the anus with your finger. That might be enough anal fun right there. But if you are getting signs and words of approval, very gently press the pad of a lubed forefinger into the anus and see how that goes. Wiggle and explore, always gingerly, slowly. You can use vibe toys around the butt hole too. Play!

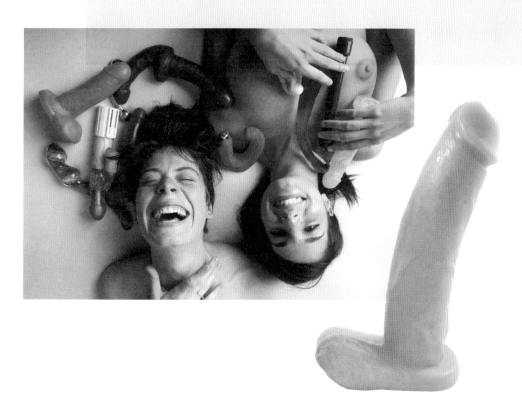

ALL HANDS ON DICK

IN PRAISE OF THE HAND JOB

"Hand jobs? Puh-lease, I gave those up after eighth grade," you might say. Maybe a hand job is the first thing you did when you touched a penis—and perhaps the first thing you did to make a guy come. But a good old-fashioned hand job never wears out its welcome. Picture a long transatlantic flight to Paris. Everyone around you is sleeping. That's the time to give your lover some nice hand-crankage under the fleecy airline blanket. Other merits of the hand job? They can offer more friction and a tighter grip than a mouth or pussy (for those who seek that). And hand jobs offer a way to feel closer to someone new. You want to get him off, but you aren't ready for oral intimacy. Just like eighth grade! Hand jobs also teach you more about the person's body, since you can see his reactions face-to-face. But the number one reason to master the hand job (aside from the fact that your sweetheart may just dig a great hand job) is: good handiwork is essential for a good blow job.

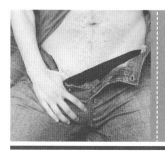

FANCY HAND MOVES FOR HIM

After you get him started, try any and all of these moves to keep him going.

Milking It

Grasp around the base and slide your hand up and off the tip. Then grab at the base and slide up again. Repeat. Like you are milking a cow. As one recipient put it, "This feels like an endless vagina!"

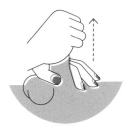

Over the Hill

Do the "Milking It" move, but then turn your hand around and come back down, tip-to base.

The Sandwich

Better than a BLT, this sandwich is 100 percent meat. Roll the penis between flattened palms like you're rolling dough. Little jiggly-roll motions are nice too. The sandwich makes a nice lead-in to the Tootsie Roll dessert.

All Thumbs

Cradle the penis with both hands, so your thumbs meet over the frenulum (that is, where the head meets the shaft on the underside). Give a gentle massage to the frenulum with both of your thumbs.

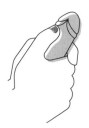

Say "Heel"

Using the heel of the hand, place it on his perineum, and with a gentle but firm touch, run it over the balls and up the shaft to the tip. Repeat as prompted.

Tootsie Roll

This one is popular with penises everywhere. Form rings around the dick with both of your hands. Your hands are stacked up, sort of like a baseball player does on a bat. Twist the rings back and forth in opposite directions. Try this with all five fingers from each hand or make the rings out of two or three fingers.

Romance a Go-Go

Remember, you don't have to limit your hand job to hand and cock alone. Bring in all those other tools, like boobs, mouth, tongue, nipple. Mmm.

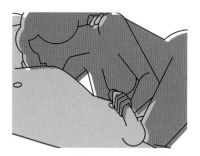

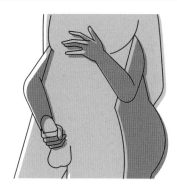

Reach Around

A perfect way to surprise him while he's doing the dishes.

Lube is the butter on the bread. So use it!

CAREFUL WITH HIS BALLS!
By all means tickle and gently fondle the balls, but don't squeeze! Unless you are explicitly told to do so.

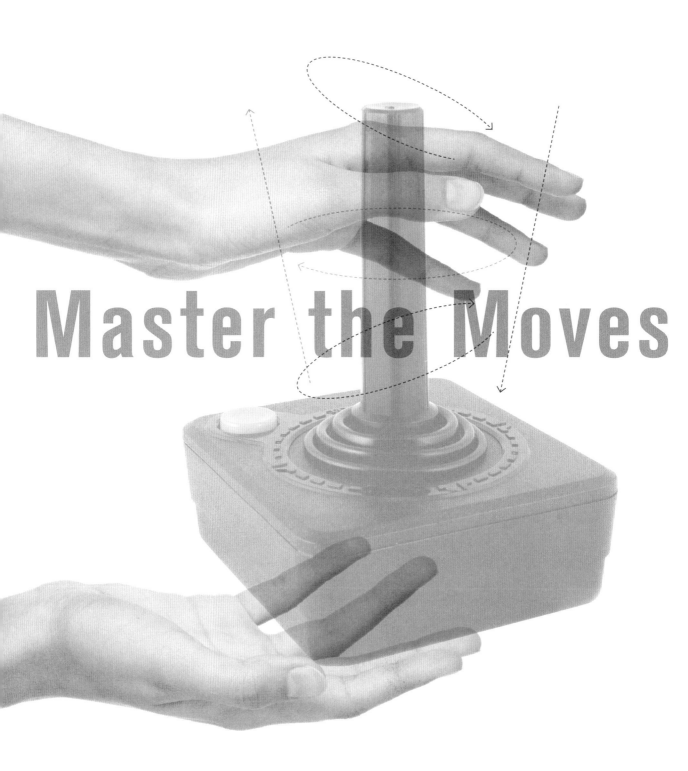

Master the Moves

MASTERING THE HAND JOB

1 Learn from a pro...him

Here's a fun and enlightening exercise. Stand behind your man while he jerks off. You really get to see his technique and rhythm from his POV. Put your hand over his hand and try to feel how much tension and squeezing there is. Take over the job and finish it yourself. Let him coach you ("Squeeze the head more" or "Go slower"). Everybody wins!

2 Add in toys

Turn your hand into a superhand with a finger vibrator. Or take a bullet vibrator (or any vibrator) and hold it against his taint, run it along the shaft, or move it around his butt hole for a new and special feeling. A masturbation sleeve is not just for him to use solo. It's like adding an extra foreskin you can slide up and down.

3 Commit to some good moves

Find a couple of moves he likes, then stick with them. When he is really getting into the rhythm of it—moaning, bucking—that's not the time to switch it up unless you want to tease a bit and delay the gushing geyser. Keep going until you want to switch to a BJ or penetration, or he comes, or you want to go knit a sweater. (That's not code—we mean really knit a sweater. It's fun to be a good lover, but quitting time is anytime you've had enough.)

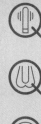

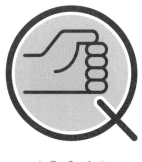

{ Q & A }

TALK TO THE HAND

{Q} "How hard do I squeeze when giving a hand job? I never know."

{A} Each cock is different. Start a generic up-and-down pumping motion and ask. "Let's work on a scale of one to ten—one being loosey-goosey and ten being tight as sex with a drinking straw. I'm calling this a five—what number should I be aiming for?" We're sure he'll oblige and enjoy this little game. This is a good feedback tool for any sexual activity you are trying to improve. As in, "If a rating one is awful and ten is fireworks, then how good does it feel when I suck your balls?"

{Q} "Boil it down for me. What's the key to a successful and rewarding hand job?"

{A} Lube. All you need is lube. Even guys who are lube-phobic when it comes to penetration probably lube up when polishing their own pipes. They might use moisturizer, which is not great because it soaks in too quickly. It also doesn't taste good if you decide to get oral, nor was it meant to go inside the body if things go that way. And moisturizer breaks down condoms. Try a water- or silicone-based brand like the ones on p. 60. That said, some guys like a dry hand job. To each his own.

{Q} "What do I do with his balls during a hand job?"

{A} Don't ignore them. Give them some pets and caresses. Every now and then, include the balls in your upstroke, with your thumb around the cock and the fingers scooping the ball sack up from underneath, gently squashing it against the shaft. (Consult cock owner and see if he approves.) Definitely massage the taint (the area between the balls and the asshole). You can feel the internal base of the penis in there. Give that area some loving. Keep in mind that testicles are fragile and hands are strong.

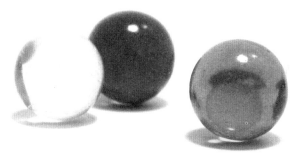

| 155

BLOW JOBS

THE JOY OF
ORAL SEX ON A GUY

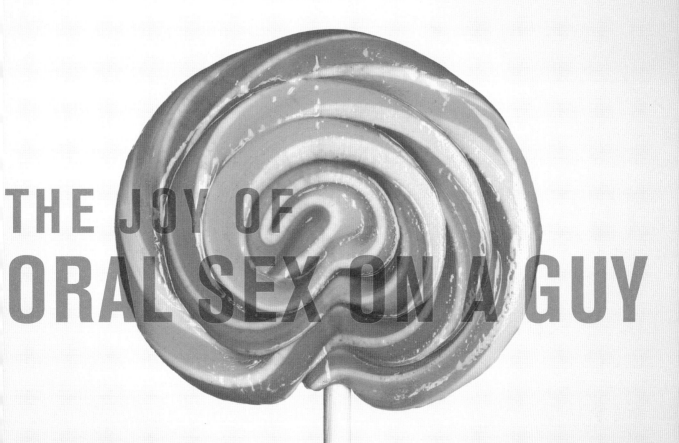

Blow jobs feel so great that some guys prefer them to intercourse. BJs are more theatrical, in some ways more intimate, and they don't make babies, which takes away a level of stress. To give a good blow job is to have great powers—the power to give pleasure and the physical control over his cock.

THE JOYSTICK IS YOURS TO PLAY WITH AS YOU SEE FIT.

You can make him come faster or slower. You can turn the strongest brute into a wiggling puddle of gratitude. So many possibilities. We want to help amp up your skills, so here are some ideas to put the O in your fellatio.

THE SECRET TO A GOOD BJ

THIS IS OUR NUMBER ONE LESSON, AND IT'S SO EASY TO LEARN:

USE YOUR HANDS A LOT.

You've got ten little sex toys with you at all times. Let them help. All the fancy hand moves we just taught you? Bring them into your BJ game. For guys, at least half the thrill is seeing a partner looking up with a hard cock in the mouth. So suck on the head, look up at your fella with a sparkle in your eye, and let your fingers do the walking. You can take up length with your hand while giving him an enveloped, deep-throat feeling. Extra bonus: you won't tire as quickly and can go all night if you want.

A MOUTH IS NOT A VAGINA

When giving head, don't try to re-create vaginal sex with your mouth. The mouth offers a whole different experience—that's why it's great! Both the mouth and the pussy have lips and get moist. But your mouth has teeth (hey, a little nibble is OK), a tongue, and an array of muscles that do things like suck and squeeze and swirl. Then once you add in the hands? Fuggedaboudit.

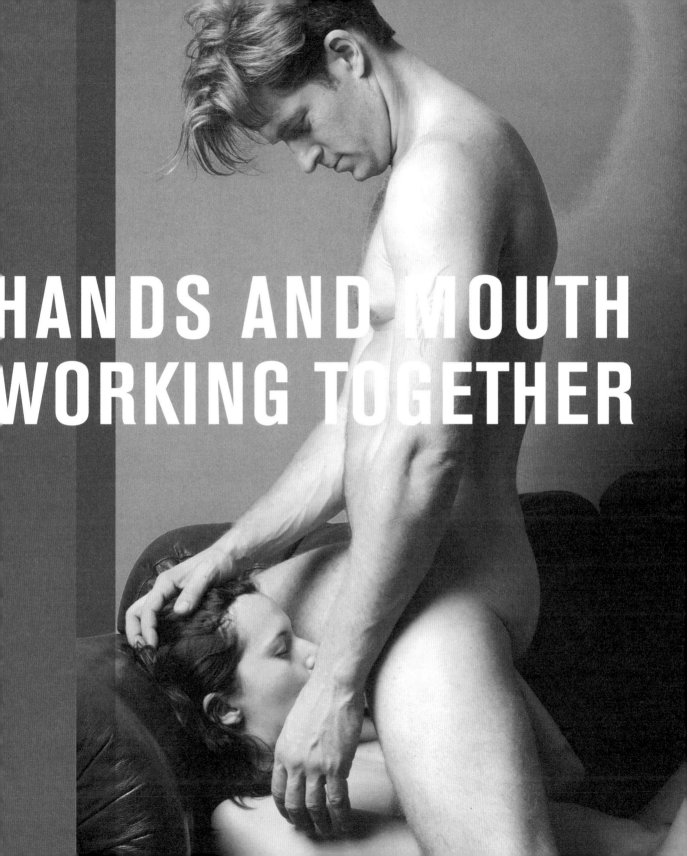

HANDS AND MOUTH
WORKING TOGETHER

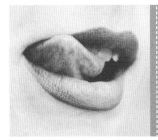

MOUTHING OFF

CONDOMS FOR COCKSUCKERS

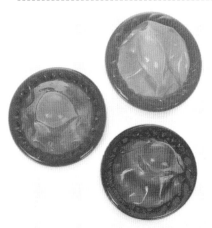

When you're in position and he gets hard, it's time to put on a condom. Oral sex is less risky than vaginal or anal sex, but you could still get HIV, herpes, chlamydia, gonorrhea, or HPV (genital warts). (See Safer Sex, p. 230.) If you're with someone new, or if your main man could be having sex with other people, use a condom and most definitely don't let him come in your mouth. You could get gonorrhea or chlamydia in your throat. The condom also acts as a cock ring, squeezing the base of the shaft. You can put a bit of lube in the receptacle tip for his pleasure.

PUT ON A CONDOM WITH YOUR MOUTH

You don't have to be a professional sex worker in Amsterdam to do this nifty trick. It's playful, so it won't feel like an interruption. This move also puts you squarely in control of the moment and your health and safety.

1 Take a condom (preferably nonlubed and flavored) out of the package. Make sure you have the correct side so the rolled-up ring will unroll correctly.

2 Put a dollop of lube in the tip, then suck the reservoir tip of the condom like it's a little baby bottle.

3 Place the condom on the head of the penis (look, no hands!) and roll it down the shaft with your mouth. You can assist in the unrolling with your hand if you need to.

4 Practice on a banana or a dildo. Or practice on your sweetie pie!

TONGUE OPTIONS

Remember that your tongue is a muscle that can swirl and change shape. You can also let the tongue be relaxed and mushy or tight and strong. There are two main ways to hold your tongue:

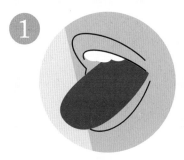

Flat for ice cream licks.

Pointy for flickering around the corona or under the balls.

SPECIAL MOUTH MOVES

Here are some suggestions to add to your routine so it's, well, less routine. Feel free to mix and match and change them to work better for you. Combine with the hand moves from p. 151, and you'll be unstoppable.

Slap Happy

Make your tongue flat and broad, open your mouth wide, and slap his cock against it.

Figure Eight

Not just for skaters. With your tongue, start at the underside of the shaft at the base and lick a figure eight up and around the shaft, back to your starting point, then down around the ball sack.

The Hummer

More powerful and earth-friendly than an SUV. You gently put your mouth around his balls and hum. Your mouth becomes the idling motor of a human vibrator.

The Twist

Twist your head as it goes up and down on his shaft, as if his cock were a barber's pole and you are tracing the spiral stripes. You can twist a lot or a little—he'll notice either way.

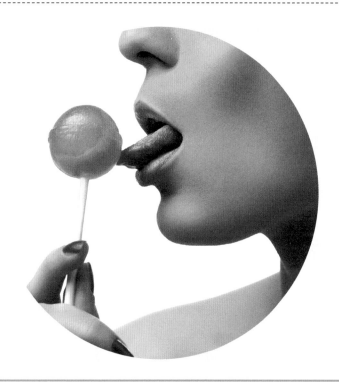

Human Cock Ring

Take two or three fingers and a thumb, and make a firm ring around the base of the shaft while you work the shaft and head with your mouth. You can also make this hand ring under the scrotum and around the base of the whole package. This will limit the blood flow out of his erection and make it last longer. If you want to free up your hand by using a real cock ring, put it on when he's semi-erect.

The Lollipop

Suck on the head of the penis and let it pop out of your mouth—complete with a fun popping noise.

GET INTO POSITION

FELLATIO HAS A BUILT-IN POWER DYNAMIC THAT CAN TIP EITHER WAY.

Like being submissive?
• Try the more cock-worshippy positions.

Want to be in complete control of your guy?
• Climb on top and express that urge.

Just want to get your sweetheart off without too much athleticism or strain?
• Find a position that allows you both to relax.

Pick one of these for starters, but by all means switch it up as you merrily go along.

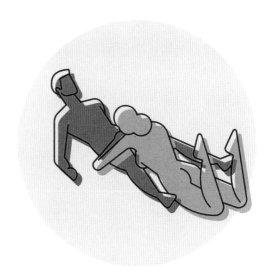

THE RECLINER

Man lies down on his back. Giver lies between his legs. Good for visuals and eye contact. Can be rough on the neck.

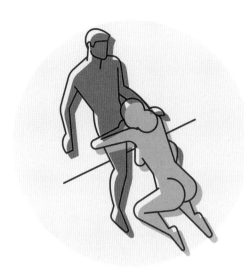

THE CONFESSIONAL

Man sits on chair, couch, or edge of bed. Giver kneels between his legs. Good for giver's neck.

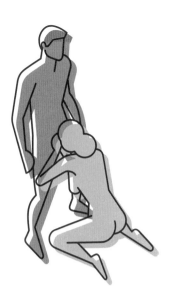

THE ELEVATOR

He stands. Giver kneels, like you'd do in an elevator. (Think Glenn Close and Michael Douglas elevator scene—pre-bunny—in *Fatal Attraction*.) Feels very subservient, which could be good or bad, depending on your mood.

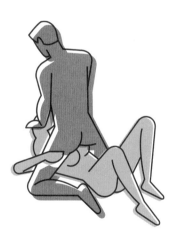

THE FACE SITTER

Giver lies on back. The man straddles giver's face and puts his cock in their mouth (a.k.a. face-fucking). This provides the blower very little control, but it's also less work. Only do this one with someone you really trust, so you don't get anxious.

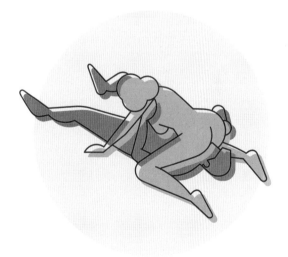

THE "HOWDY!"

Man lies on his back. The giver straddles him upside-down, with giver's feet by the man's head. Man gets up-close view of the ass—he can finger the asshole and tender parts or return the favor with some 69.

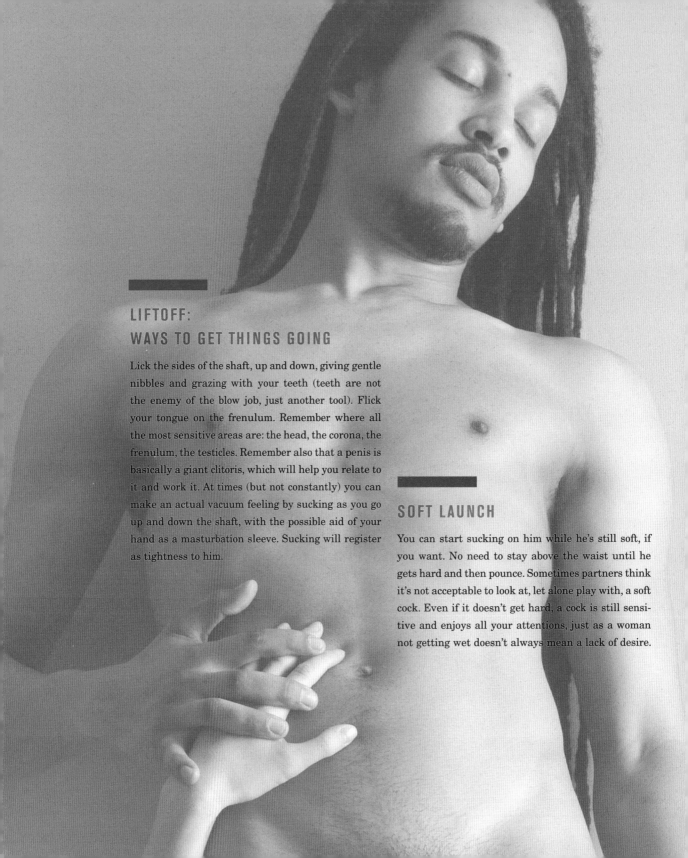

LIFTOFF:
WAYS TO GET THINGS GOING

Lick the sides of the shaft, up and down, giving gentle nibbles and grazing with your teeth (teeth are not the enemy of the blow job, just another tool). Flick your tongue on the frenulum. Remember where all the most sensitive areas are: the head, the corona, the frenulum, the testicles. Remember also that a penis is basically a giant clitoris, which will help you relate to it and work it. At times (but not constantly) you can make an actual vacuum feeling by sucking as you go up and down the shaft, with the possible aid of your hand as a masturbation sleeve. Sucking will register as tightness to him.

SOFT LAUNCH

You can start sucking on him while he's still soft, if you want. No need to stay above the waist until he gets hard and then pounce. Sometimes partners think it's not acceptable to look at, let alone play with, a soft cock. Even if it doesn't get hard, a cock is still sensitive and enjoys all your attentions, just as a woman not getting wet doesn't always mean a lack of desire.

GET YOUR PH.D. IN HUMMERS

1 Use your mouth creatively

Hold your mouth and his cock still, but let your tongue swirl all around it inside. Hold some hot tea or cold water in your mouth for a few seconds and then get oral. Or rub his cock over your lips and face.

2 Add toys

All of the hand-job toys we suggested are also fun for fellating: cock ring, finger vibrator, masturbation sleeve. You can also hold a vibrator to your cheek or jaw while going downtown. Then your warm, moist mouth vibrates for a new sensation.

3 Play ball! (or with them)

Ball play is easier with the mouth because you can be gentler, and it's easier to control the amount of pressure. Remember how sensitive his balls are. Kiss lightly—enjoy the alive nature of the scrotal skin as it scrunches up and swirls. Speaking of swirls, you can spiral your tongue around his whole ball sack. Or just let his balls rest on your face and lips. By the way, balls in your mouth or resting on your face is called "tea-bagging"—not to be confused with what Queen Elizabeth does with friends and heads of state at 4 P.M. every day.

4 Deep throat

Deep-throating is when you take the cock extra far into your mouth and even into your throat. Most of the cock nerves are in the head, so deep-throating doesn't do as much for the guy physically as it does visually. It takes the power dynamics of BJs a step further. Only do this with a partner you really trust.

ADDING IN SOME ANAL

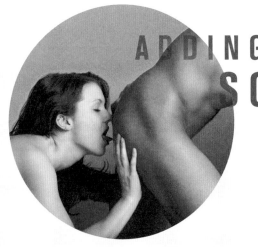

Some guys beg for anal play. They know about all of the nerve endings in the anus and the power of the prostate. Others aren't as experienced. Try a conversation ahead of time and ask him how he feels about anal play. If his answer is something like "I'm intrigued" or "I tried it but didn't like it, but I'd give it another go," you're golden. If somehow you forgot to have that talk between the taxi and the bedroom, send out some feelers (of the pinkie variety) and see how he responds. Here's one (but certainly not the only) path to giving him backdoor pleasure.

RIM JOB RECIPE

• Time this for when he's fresh out of the shower.

• Start by licking and sucking on the testicles.

• If he isn't freshened up, cut open a condom or use non-microwaveable plastic wrap as a barrier for oral fun. Or else just skip the rim job and keep it digital from here (as in fingers).

• Lick the taint—it's not a big leap from taint to butt hole once you are in the neighborhood.

• Make sure everything is wet. Add lube if necessary.

• Use broad ice cream strokes on the butt hole while working your hand on his dick.

• Gently massage the anus with the flat pad of your index finger. Let the massage evolve into a probe inward—gentle and slow. This works well when he is turned on from BJ action.

• If that meets with approval, lube up and gently put your finger about two inches in and curve it toward his belly—there lies the prostate, which enjoys some nice finger stroking.

• Or skip the rim job entirely and just give him a little pinkie while sucking his cock. It practically guarantees fireworks.

TITTY SEX!

It's like a hand job except with your breasts (big ones not required). Using lube will make everything better (per usual!). It's easier for him to thrust his cock than for you to thrust your chest. You can lie on your back and have him straddle you, with his penis between your boobs. Or you can kneel and face him while he sits on the edge of the bed (depending on everyone's height). If you are small-breasted, you can use your hands to smush your boobs together on his cock. Add as much hand action as you need. This event is very much about the visual effect, so make sure he has a good view.

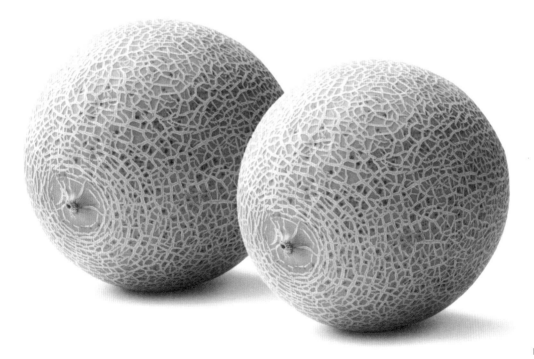

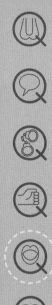

{ Q & A }

BJ Qs

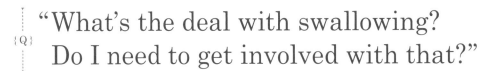

{Q} ## "What's the deal with swallowing? Do I need to get involved with that?"

{A} It's one of the age-old questions of sexual etiquette. The question is not, "What does a nice girl do?" but, "What makes you comfortable and keeps you connected to your desire?" It's your choice. No need to make excuses, and no need to have regrets. Swallowing his semen is no big deal from a health perspective. Some men tell you they are about to come, and then you can just swallow (do two or three gulps with your throat so you make sure you get it all). Or shut the back of your throat till he's done and then swallow. If you choose not to swallow, why not play up the theatricality and have a big finale? Then you can both watch his money shot. Let him come on your face, your neck, your chest—wherever's fun. But don't get semen in your eyes (just close 'em at the last minute!), because it can cause an infection.

{Q} ## "My sweetie can't stand it when I touch him after he comes. What's up with that?"

{A} Many guys' dicks get super sensitive after they come. It's as if their steel-hard love unit turns to fragile porcelain. When a second ago they were begging, "Harder, faster, deeper," they suddenly cry, "Oh, God, stop, don't touch it." Be ready to shift gears and stop what you were doing just a second ago. Chances are you feel the same way after great oral sex.

{Q} "I have a partner who needs very rough stimulation to 'feel anything,' as he puts it. He masturbates very roughly and likes me to scrape his dick with my teeth. Can we increase his sensitivity to gentler touches?"

{A} Lots of people visit Babeland and tell us this. They say it is the only way they can get off. And that may be true. There are so many ways to get off if you take the time and patience to experiment (on yourself, on your partner). So he could learn new tricks, but if he's happy, there is no real need. Gentle touch isn't better than rough play. That said, he's a great candidate for a vibrator. Try working a Silver Bullet along his shaft and under his balls. Or try taking a break from sex for a while and see if he is more sensitive after some time off.

{Q} "How can I tame my gag reflex? I mean, I can't breathe when that thing's in my mouth."

{A} We are biologically programmed to gag when something tickles the back of the throat. The uvula, that pendulum that dangles from the roof of your mouth in the back (and is drawn into the mouths of all the Muppets), helps set off the gag reflex. Here are some easy steps to help avoid the gaggage:

• Try to aim him down toward your tongue side, not up toward your roof side.
• Relax your cheeks, tongue, and jaw. Open the back of your throat by saying "ah," like the doctor asks you to do when poking in a tongue depressor.
• Even easier: don't take his cock in so deep you gag. Let your hand on his dick extend the tunnel you make with your mouth.
• Breathe, baby, breathe. In general, try to take in air when on the "out" thrust, when the cock is out of the mouth. Breathe through your nose as much as possible. Dirty talk can be a way to take a break and catch your breath. Or shake things up by kissing other parts of his body.

{Q} "My boyfriend's jizz is bitter. Can he change it?"

{A} Yes. For example, smoking or eating spicy foods can make semen bitter. Meat eaters will taste different from vegetarians. Eating more fruit will sweeten his come. Specifics? Try pineapple, celery, and parsley, and drink lots of water. Stay away from garlic, onions, broccoli, and, most of all, asparagus!

GOING DOWN
EAT YOUR HEART OUT

There's a reason women have another set of lips below the belt (two sets, actually). Those lips are for kissing ... and licking and sucking and generally worshipping.

THE HUMAN TONGUE IS ONE OF NATURE'S GREAT SEX TOOLS.

It can be soft or hard, it generates extra lube, it has muscles but no bones, and it bends. Ounce for ounce, it's the strongest muscle in the human body. Seems a waste not to give a girl pleasure with it.

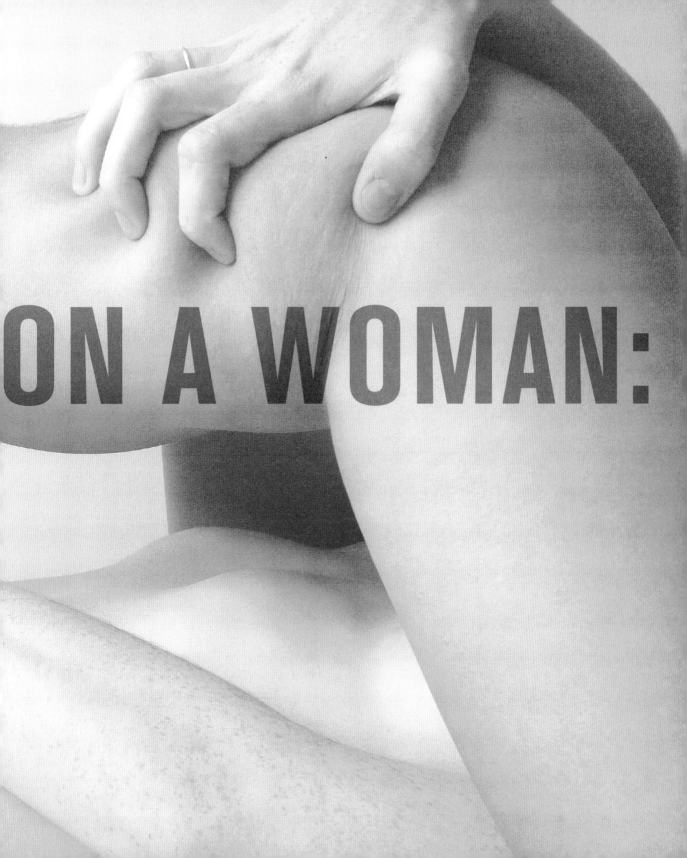

ON A WOMAN:

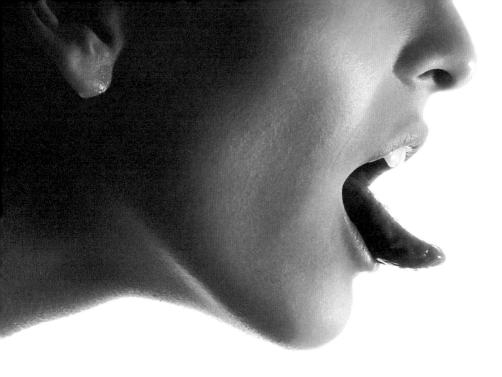

FUCK A WOMAN WITH YOUR MOUTH

Like everything else in this life, great oral sex takes passion and practice (and passion for practice!). Here are several ways to maximize her pleasure.

WARM HER UP

Introduce yourself to her cooch. Put your hand on her vulva and touch her thighs. Go European and give two or three friendly hello kisses.

CHECKING FOR FEEDBACK

It might be hard for you to talk, though if you moan and growl and hum, you make your face into a vibrator! If you're wondering if she likes what you're doing, stop and ask a dirty question. "Is your kitty purring?"

Since you are right there, notice how her vulva is getting engorged and if her parts are reddening. See if she is pushing and bucking and clutching. Listen for coaching from above. ("Eeek, softer!" "Mmmm. Yes." And the like.)

BUILD IT AND SHE MAY COME ...

Build up the intensity level gradually. Once you're in high gear, use your whole face. Bury yourself in her muff. Make your tongue pointy and strong, and push it in as far as possible. Use your nose for more pressure. Not only does this feel good physically, it lets her know you are really into her taste and smell. We like to say: if your eyelids aren't sticky, you're not doing it right. Find some movement she likes and repeat it rhythmically. Once you are in that intense rhythmic place, it is NOT the time to mix it up with new moves. If it's working, keep going!

YOU SUCK (IN A GOOD WAY)

Sucking feels good for a woman, too. Sucking on her clit is like a gentle mini blow job for her. Pull the clit into your mouth and create suction while swirling with your tongue.

G-SPOTTING AND SQUIRTING

You can try to reach the G-spot with your tongue, but fingers and toys can probably reach it better and stroke it harder. (See the guide on p. 144 for manual pleasuring.) Insert two fingers while licking her clit and press her G-spot below while your mouth is pushing from above. We are always pleased to see hand and mouth skills combined. Finger-fucking and oral combined are like the lesbian missionary position. A tried-and-true classic that's good for everybody.

GIVE IT ALL YOU'VE GOT

Use your hands to feel her body, her ass, her nipples; wrap your arms around her hips and press above her pubic mound to expose and tighten the clit and put pressure on her inner muscles. If you are using your hand to fuck her while going down on her, get fancy by adding a backdoor pinkie to the mix.

TOYS!

If she wants deeper penetration, try your fingers or a dildo. There are some lovely curved G-spotting toys for the occasion. If she likes outside sensation more than penetration, grab a vibe and buzz all around her vulva—while you lick or rest.

TONGUE-ERCISES

The people you love and the people you lick will thank you if you strengthen your tongue, so it can work like an anaconda of *amore*. **Try some of these while watching TV or driving a car. (If other drivers see you, just smile and wave.) Avoid doing these on boring dates or in business meetings.**

NOSIES: Stick out your tongue and curve it up to your nose. Can you touch the tip of your nose with the tip of your tongue? (Do two sets of three.)

CHINSIES: Stick out your tongue and curve it down to your chin. See how far down on your chin you can reach. (Do two sets of three.)

TOOTHPICKS: Open your mouth and pretend there's a toothpick holding it open, just behind your teeth. Keep your tongue inside and slowly run the tip of your tongue up and down this imaginary toothpick. Go up and down five times. Then, keeping your mouth open, do the same movement as fast as you can, fluttering the tip of your tongue top to bottom. (Flutter fast for a slow count of five.)

LIZARDS: This exercise is for side-to-side strengthening and motor skills. Part your lips a little and let your tongue peek out. Without touching your lips, run your tongue from the leftcorner to the right corner along the lip line. (Do two sets of five.)

CRUSHERS: Take a small piece of candy like an M&M or a Skittle (if you are off sweets, a single Cheerio will do) and place it on the tip of your tongue. Then, with your tongue, place the candy on the roof of your mouth, on the ridge just above and behind your front teeth. Press the candy steadily with your tongue until it crushes or dissolves. This will give your tongue strength and endurance.

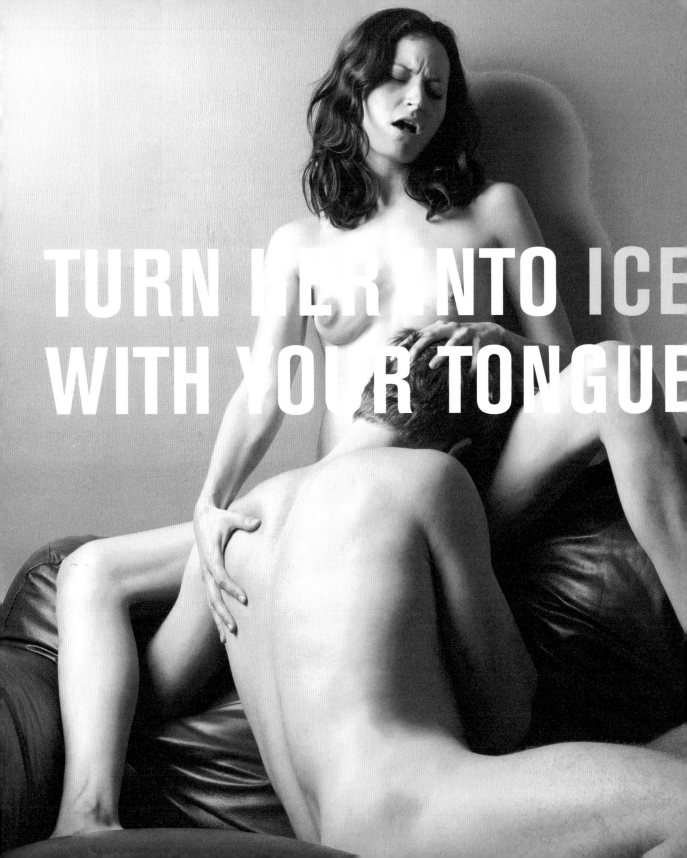

TURN HER INTO ICE
WITH YOUR TONGUE

CREAM

Remember that your tongue can be wide and flat or strong and pointy (among other possibilities—but those are two ends of the spectrum). Start your dive with a wide and flat tongue. Lick her from perineum to pubes with big, broad strokes that will wake up all the nerves.

LICK HER SLOWLY AND LUSCIOUSLY,

like her V is the world's tastiest ice cream cone, three scoops high. (Add in flavored lube to make her dessert-ier if you want.) Big, soft licks from bottom to top. If she's not crazy about the vag licks, just concentrate on the clit with a nice, big, fat, soft tongue.

TAKE YOUR POSITION

HERE ARE SOME IDEAS FOR HER SATISFACTION.

The Recliner and the Little Prayer are good for starting with a new partner. And feel free to switch your position as you go!

RECEIVING AS WELL AS GIVING

Being a great giver is, well, awesome. But there's also some thought, skill, and effort involved in being a good receiver of pleasure. Do you get self-conscious? Do you quiet down like a clam? The person in bed with you is working their little heart (or tongue) out and they deserve to know if you're enjoying it. In fact, some positive feedback will probably get your sweetie hotter, which will inspire more tongue work, which will get you hotter. This is not the time to act mysterious or let worries take over ("Do they notice my thigh mole?"). Show some appreciation! Give some feedback—a couple of "Oh yeahs" when they get you in your good spot, for example. If you're sinking into the experience and talking is tough, rolling hips, moaning, and spreading your legs farther apart are all great ways of expressing your pleasure without words. But if you do have something to say, speak up! Don't leave some good-hearted pussy eater painting the wrong side of the fence because you feel shy. Touching your partner is a sweet way to connect. If there's a head in your lap, stroke its hair. It's a way of saying thank you.

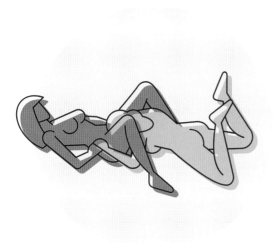

THE RECLINER (FOR HER)

The classic cunnilingus pose is when she reclines and you lie on your stomach with your head between her open legs. And that's a good one. It creates nice visuals for her and makes for easy eye contact. The only downside is that your neck doesn't like it after a while.

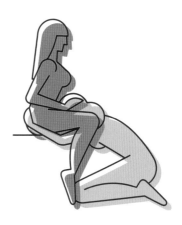

THE LITTLE PRAYER

You're kneeling at the edge of the bed while she sits or lies back, facing you with legs open.

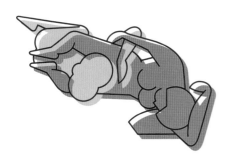

THE S CURVE

She lies on her right side in a semifetal position. You lie on your left side facing her, farther down, with your head to her muff. The two of you form a big S from above. Great for the neck. Bad for eye contact. Can be a little awkward for her top leg that's over your ear—but you can work it out.

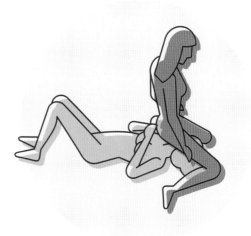

THE FACE SITTER

The lickee straddles the face of the licker, giving the lickee lots of fun control. Good visuals. Make sure the person on the bottom can breathe—if she starts slapping at you, get off! It can be hard to come while holding yourself up. Try placing your hands on the wall at the edge or top of the bed, and coming will come easier.

THE PROS AND CONS OF 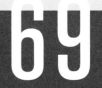69

Sixty-nine is a sex position that allows simultaneous oral sex. Two people get head-to-toe and toe-to-head like a human yin-yang symbol. Some folks love this maneuver, others do not. Here's why ...

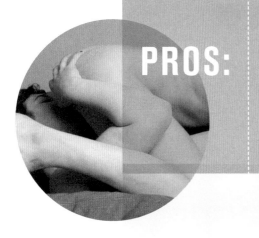

PROS:

- It's show-offy and fun just for stunt value.
- If one person getting oral is great, then 69 is double the greatness.
- Fun for mutual pleasuring.

- Very fair in terms of master/servant power dynamics.
- Gives you a good view you rarely get otherwise.
- Helpful angle for deep-throating too.

For some people, this equal-opportunity position means no opportunity to concentrate and enjoy. It can be hard to enjoy the getting if you are busy giving.

Can be awkward physically.

Some folks miss the eye contact, 'cause all you see are tender parts and butt.

ALTERNATIVE POSITION #34.5: Most people do 69 with one person on their back and the other straddling above. It might be better if you both got on your sides. Another good adaptation is what we call "34.5," where one person reclines and the other person crouches with knees to one side of the reclined person's head. Or straddling the reclined person's head. The top person performs oral coming down from above, while the prone person just kicks back and enjoys. You get the groovy angle but half the action. Everyone can concentrate. Then if you want, switcheroo for fairness!

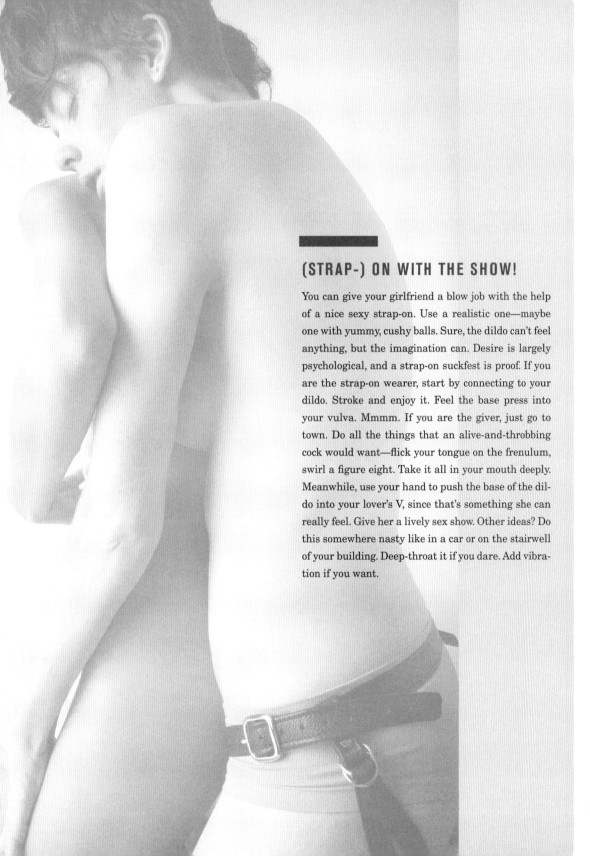

(STRAP-) ON WITH THE SHOW!

You can give your girlfriend a blow job with the help of a nice sexy strap-on. Use a realistic one—maybe one with yummy, cushy balls. Sure, the dildo can't feel anything, but the imagination can. Desire is largely psychological, and a strap-on suckfest is proof. If you are the strap-on wearer, start by connecting to your dildo. Stroke and enjoy it. Feel the base press into your vulva. Mmmm. If you are the giver, just go to town. Do all the things that an alive-and-throbbing cock would want—flick your tongue on the frenulum, swirl a figure eight. Take it all in your mouth deeply. Meanwhile, use your hand to push the base of the dildo into your lover's V, since that's something she can really feel. Give her a lively sex show. Other ideas? Do this somewhere nasty like in a car or on the stairwell of your building. Deep-throat it if you dare. Add vibration if you want.

CUNNILINGUS Qs

{Q} "I love going down on my sweetheart, but she has a hard time coming. How can I make it happen for her?"

{A} Building tension is necessary and sometimes takes a while. No clocks allowed! If you're onto something good, do it for a bit, then back off the intensity, do it again, then back off and so on. Getting her close and then deliberately backing away will get her to a place where the orgasm will become inevitable. Rhythm is sexier than random licks, and finding the right pressure for her is key. Tongue on clit plus fingers inside works for a lot of people. If you both enjoy it whether she comes or not, this may help her come. Ironic and true.

"My girl wants a rim job, but I'm a backdoor novice. How do I get started?"

For tongue-to-butt-hole pleasuring, the best bet is to wash up first. But if that doesn't happen, use a barrier (a dental dam, a condom cut open, nonmicrowaveable plastic wrap). Never bring butt bacteria to her pussy, as it can cause infection. If she's showered, and the rim job is either the main event or the dessert after pussy licking is done, then go ahead and contact the skin directly. Use your tongue to trace swirls around her A-hole until you feel it relax and even pucker out a bit. Just stay on the outside, or add an amply lubed finger or toy if she yearns for penetration.

"Can I use whipped cream when I go down on my girlfriend?"

Yum! Sounds delectable. The only danger here is that unfortunately, sugar is the key ingredient in a surefire recipe for a yeast infection. The bacterial balance of the puss needs to be maintained just so, or things get mighty itchy. Your safest bet for a tasty treat is flavored lube. But that's really not the same, is it? If you do use whipped cream, try a sugar-free brand, which won't have the sugar but may have some other irritants, depending on how sensitive the person is. With any food, keep it on the surface and avoid creamy tongue pokes into the vag. And all oils are bad for latex, so keep that in mind.

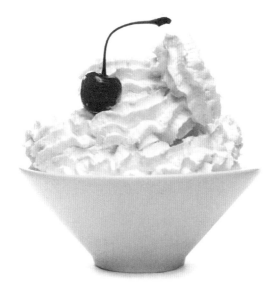

CHAPTER 6

STICKING IT IN:

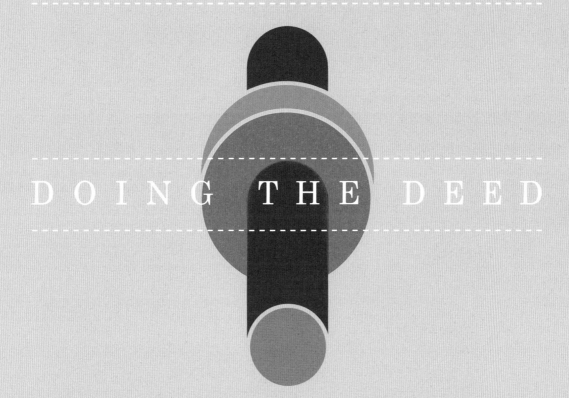

DOING THE DEED

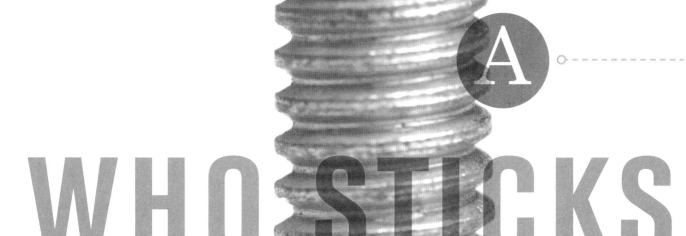

A

WHO STICKS

Sex is more than just penetration. For some couples, "going all the way" means oral or manual pleasuring. For others, anal sex is the real ticket. And for many, **PENETRATION CAN BE WITH HAND OR TONGUE OR COCK OR TOY OR ELBOW** if that's what feels right. We just wanted to remind you that "sex" and "sticking it in" deserve broad definition. And we're just the broads to remind you.

WHAT WHERE?

B

SEX: A BIG FUCKING DEAL?

If you have sex with someone, then see the person at a party five years later, you will not be able to stop yourself from thinking, "Oh my God, I did it with this person. Oh my God." And then you'll politely ask how the person's job is going. Sex can put you on a new plane of closeness. Sex—good sex—means two people making each other feel so good that they totally live in the moment. If all goes well, it's impossible to think about why you're mad at your mom or what you need to get done at the office while you're fucking. It's a gift. It's a joy. It's an exciting, entertaining escape from the everyday. That's why they call it "the poor man's opera."

Going "all the

GETTING CLOSER TO DOING THE DEED

At Babeland, we have a very generous idea of what "doing it" is, but our culture puts penis-in-vagina sex on a pedestal all its own as the ultimate "doing it." This leaves out lesbian and gay sex, and leaves some straight people wondering just what constitutes a queer home run. That said, we know that for most straight people having intercourse is a notable line to cross. And when it's good, it's very, very good: mutual pleasure, parts fitting together just so, maybe even orgasms at almost the same moment. And when you want it, you want it. Sometimes you get that itch that only a good shag will scratch. On the flip side, bad fucking (straight or gay) sucks: it can feel isolating if you're not into it, or mechanical if it's not the right person, time, or place. Thinking about whether or not you're ready to do the deed (ideally, before you're in the bed, naked) is a sound idea. If you haven't already vetted this lover, here are three key questions you may want to ask yourself before you go any further.

Do I trust this person emotionally?

It's very important to decide if you feel safe from harm. Has this person treated other lovers well in the past? A good indicator: Do they talk about exes with respect? Does this person seem solicitous of you? Do they ask if you've had enough to eat or if you're warm enough? Does this person make you feel good about yourself? If the answer to any of these is no, do not pass "go."

Have you worked out your birth control? And safer sex?

Was your partner ready to enter your pearly gates without talking about this? That's not cool. Even if you're on the pill, you still need a condom and certainly a discussion. A simple "Do you have a condom?" is a good start. (See more on safe sex on p. 230).

What do I want out of this encounter, emotionally?

If this is a one-night stand on a business trip, then the emotional stakes are pretty low. If this is a person you want as a girlfriend or boyfriend, do you think sex (or sex too soon) will change things? Maybe not, but take a mental moment to ask if doing this will change the way this person treats you—for better or worse? If sex is a big deal to you, then it might feel right to proceed slowly. One friend suggests that if you don't feel comfortable calling the person the next day, maybe it's too soon.

PENETRATION:
NOT JUST TAB A IN SLOT B

If God really wanted all straight sex to be in the missionary position, the penis would come equipped with those fluttering rabbit ears you see on sex toys or the glans of the clit would be inside the vagina. But fortunately there's a built-in challenge: figuring out how to be a good lover, or how to be good in bed as a couple. And while we don't know what's right for every single couple, we know some basic sexual positions—perfect for fucking with penises or strap-ons—that please a lot of people. These positions are written from the point of view of a female receiver, but if you're a gal using a strap-on you can switch roles. Just because you've been getting it all night doesn't mean you can't turn around and dish it out.

GO WITH THE FLOW

If you are having a quickie before your in-laws come over, there might not be enough time to change positions. Fine. But in general, it's fun and rewarding to change it up once or twice or eight times during sex. Your arms get tired, you want a better view, you're simply getting bored. Or maybe one of you is about to come but you want to delay the explosion. So switch it up! Sexual positions are loaded with power dynamics, when you think about it. (And you might as well think about it.) For instance, the person on top is pinning the other down and controlling the thrusts. Sometimes one person is more exposed and vulnerable. So it can be fun to take turns being in charge. The following pages are filled with positions you might enjoy, if you're not already enjoying. And anyway, when you go out dancing, you don't do the same move all night, do you?

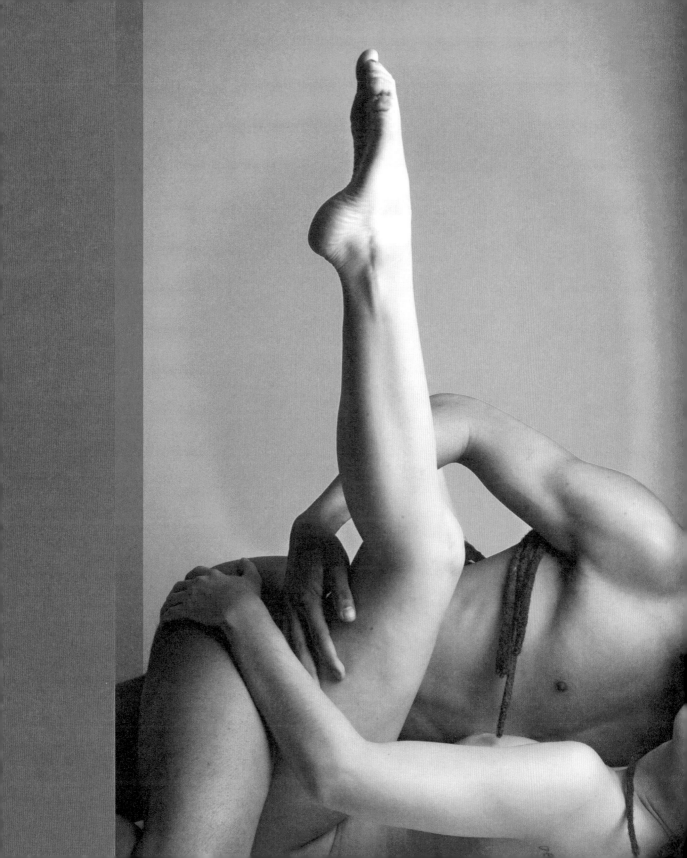

MISSIONARY

Description:

You're on your back with your legs parted. Your partner is on top, facing you.

Pros:

- It's a classic for a reason.
- You can talk, kiss, bite, and make eye contact.
- Genital contact is nice and deep.
- You can grind your pelvis against your partner for indirect clit stimulation.

Cons:

- You can't control the thrusting as much, and you're somewhat pinned down.
- Your partner can get tired from holding their torso up, like in a push-up. Or else your partner's weight is resting on you, which can get squashy.

Notes:

Since your arms are free, you can clench the headboard, which looks sexy and gives you a new kind of leverage. Your can rub your sweetie's shoulders, tickle or scratch their back, grab your partner's ass, play with their ears and hair. Your legs are free to spread wide or wrap around their waist for even deeper penetration. You can bend your knees and rest your feet on your partner's thighs or butt for a superdeep plunge and more thrust control.

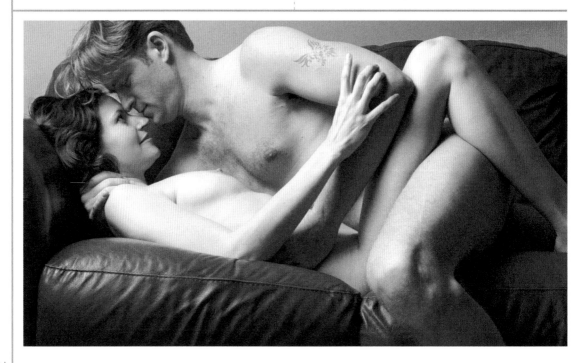

Missionary Variations:

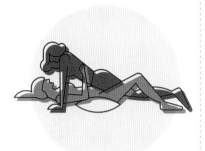

ASSISTED MISSIONARY

Sounds like a government project (we wish!). Put a pillow or two under your butt or under your lower back. This will tilt your pelvis up to better match the natural angle of the penis or dildo. This is also nice if you suffer from back pain.

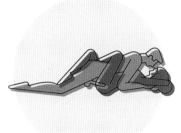

POWER UP

Add hands-free vibration to the fun. The wearable We vibe, which stimulates the clit and the G-spot and is made to be worn during intercourse, or a vibrating cock ring can provide the clit stimulation that the missionary position sometimes denies.

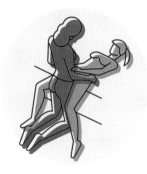

LIFE ON THE EDGE

Lie down on your back at the edge of the bed, with your thighs and legs dangling off. Bend your knees and put your feet on the ground. Your partner stands or kneels between your legs and enters you. Your partner gets a great view and control of a deep thrust. You get to kick back and enjoy.

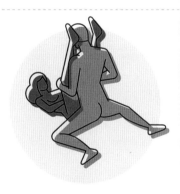

BUTT LIFT

Put your ankles on your partner's shoulders. This will lift your butt in the air. Your partner can hold your butt or your legs, and can kiss and massage your feet. Your partner has total control over the thrusting. Not great for stimulating the clit.

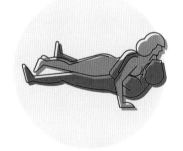

LEG REVERSAL

Hold your legs straight and together while the penetrative partner opens up their legs around yours. It takes a little more work to get the penis or dildo into the V, but then it's a nice tight feeling.

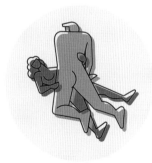

THE SCISSORS

You and your partner are making a scissor shape, with your partner's leg between one of yours and the other outside it. Lots of pressure on your mons makes this position a cut above.

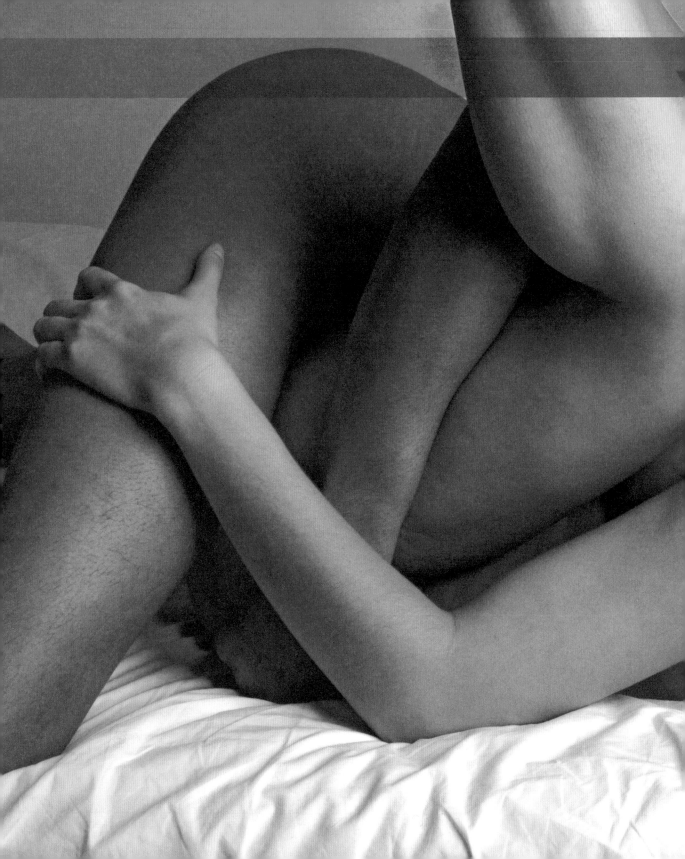

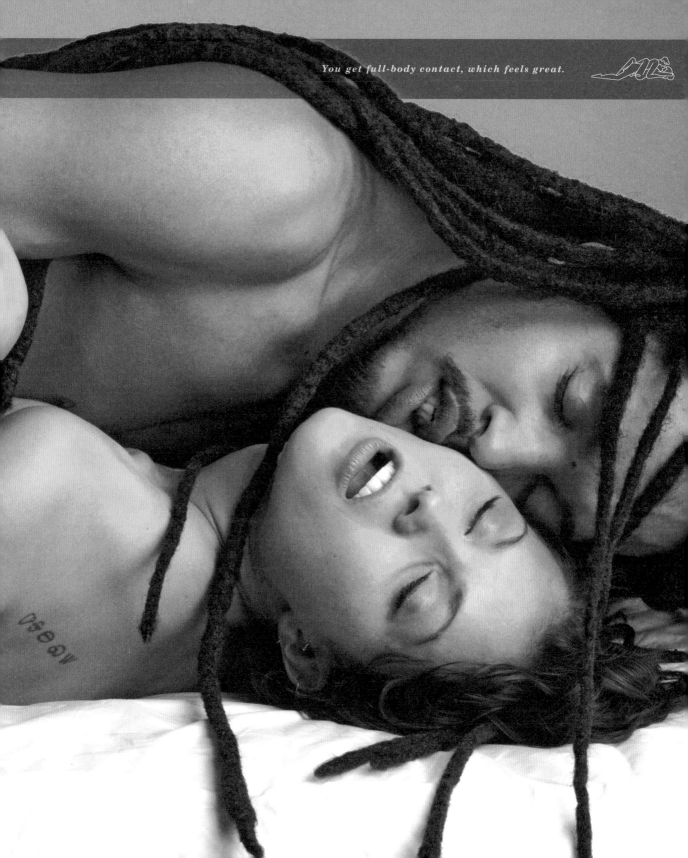

You get full-body contact, which feels great.

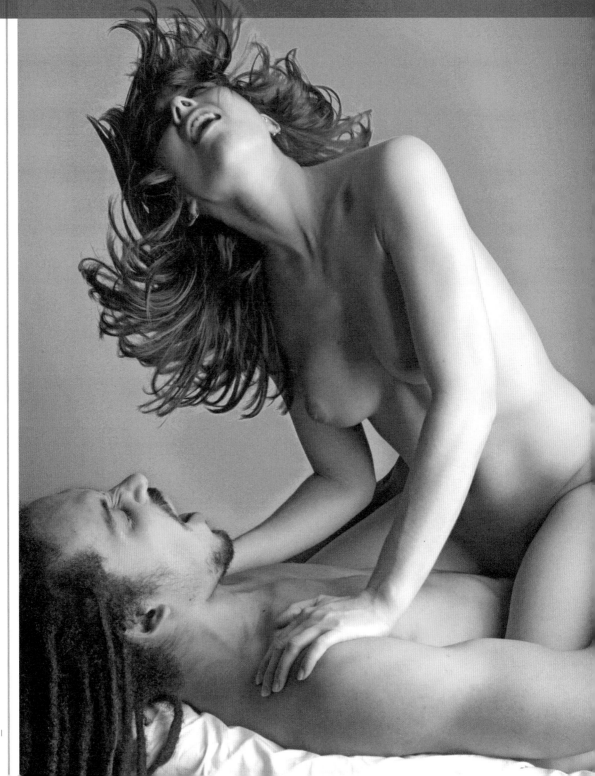

COWGIRL

Description:

Partner lies on their back. You straddle your partner on your knees. As in, "Ride 'em, Cowgirl!" You can lean on your hands to hold your weight up, or just stay up on your knees.

Pros:

- Gives you total control of depth and movement.
- Great for grinding your pelvis against your partner for clit happiness. (The more you lean forward, the better the grind.)
- Your partner gets a fantastic full-frontal view.
- You can talk and kiss and make eye contact.
- If you lean forward, your partner can suck on your nipples.

Cons:

- Your partner is pinned down and can't control depth or movement much, but gets the chance to rest.

Notes:

Your partner's hands are free to grab the headboard or touch your breasts. You can take your honey's wrists and hold them down to make clear who's the boss. In hetero sex, this position often helps the woman come sooner (or at all) and the man come later. How far forward or back you lean will change the angle and the way it feels. You can lie forward on top of your partner if you need to rest or want to feel more skin on skin.

Cowgirl Variations:

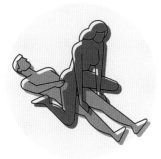

REVERSE COWGIRL

Kneel and straddle your partner, facing the other direction. You can put your arms in front of you and lean on your partner's knees. Or you can arch and lean back on your arms, behind you. This does not allow easy eye contact, but you get a lot of control.

THE FLYING BUTTRESS

This is for show-offs. Your partner is on top but facing away from you, head at your feet. Entry can be difficult from this angle. You can tilt your pelvis up to help the cause. For some, this is enjoyable. For others, it requires too much flexibility.

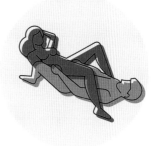

LIMBO LIKE ME

If you are flexible enough, lean back so your head is between your partner's ankles. Then your partner holds your hips to control the thrusting. This helps the cock hit the G-spot. Anybody's free hand (or vibe!) can rub the clit.

DOGGY STYLE

Description:

Doggies and most mammals do it this way. Really, this is even more of a classic than missionary. You get on all fours (leaning on your hands or your forearms) and your partner kneels behind you, grasps your hips, and enters you from behind. You may need to tilt your butt way up to make entry easy.

Pros:

- Amazing ass view for your partner, who can watch as the cock or dildo goes in and out of your V.
- Gives a tighter fit than facing positions.
- Feels delightfully naughty.
- Positions cock or dildo well for G-spot stimulation.

Cons:

- Not that much skin contact.
- No eye contact.
- No clitoral stimulation.
- If the penis or dildo is big, it can bump your cervix. (Easy to fix by backing off.)

Notes:

This position really feels like your partner is mounting and dominating you like an animal. Your partner has much more physical control. The power dynamics aren't subtle, and they can be fun. You can use one or both of your free hands to rub or vibe your clit. If you get tired, you can lean your chest forward on a pile of pillows (and maybe even stick a pillow between your legs to hump for clit fun). You can reach down between your legs and caress your partner's parts. Your partner can use one or two free hands to rub your clit and boobs, massage your back, grab a handful of hair, or spank your sweet ass.

Doggy Style Variations:

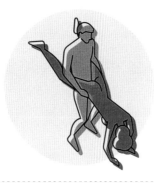

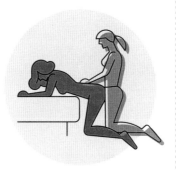

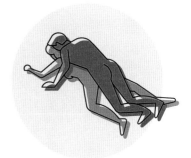

RAISED DOGGY

Your partner kneels or stands behind you and enters you. Your thighs can be apart with your partner's thighs inside yours. Whichever feels better. If your partner's a strong brute, they can (after penetration) lift and hold one or both of your legs—like a sexy wheelbarrow.

SUPPORTED DOGGY

You kneel by the side of the bed, facing it and bracing your arms against the mattress. Your partner kneels behind you. All the fun of regular doggy, but with solid support.

TIRED DOGGY

You lie face down with one or two pillows under your pelvis, so your butt tilts up. Your partner lies on top of you and enters you from behind with legs either between or outside of yours. You have little control, but it sure is restful!

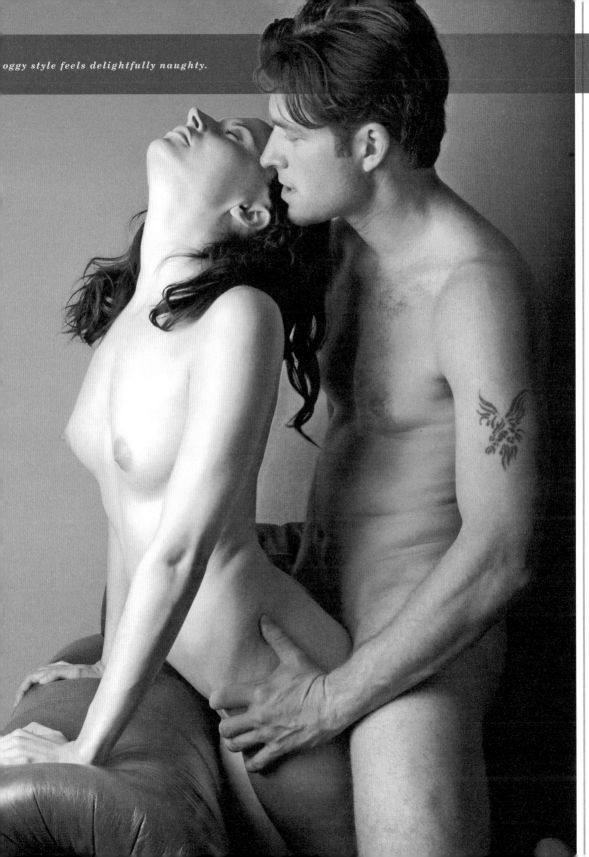

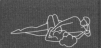

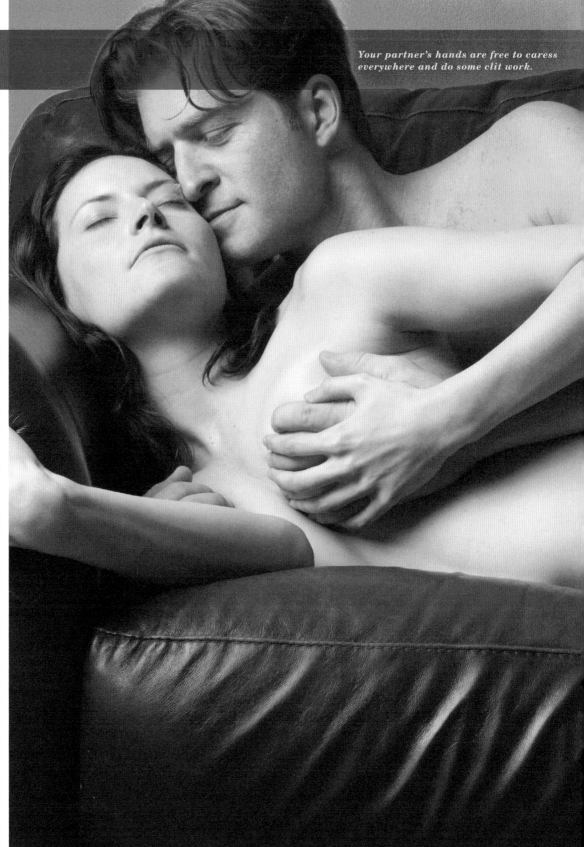

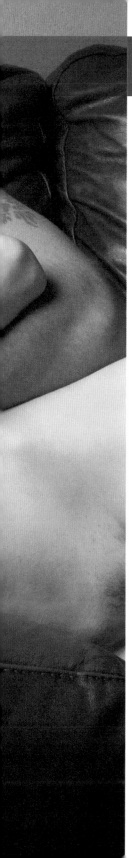

Position:

SIDE-BY-SIDE

Description:

You and your partner lie on your sides, facing the same direction, with you in front. Your partner's knees tuck into the backs of your knees. Your basic spooning position, with the added spice of penetration.

Pros:

- Relaxing! Easy! This is a great one if you're pregnant, or if you have a lusciously large belly.
- Your partner can kiss your earlobes, neck, and shoulders. You—or your partner—can rub or vibe your clit.
- Lots of skin-to-skin contact.

Cons:

- Can't exactly thrust wildly.
- May be too mellow for some.

Notes:

Your partner controls the strokes in and out, but you can tilt your butt to your favorite angle.

Side-by-Side Variations:

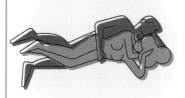

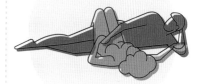

THE SIDE ROLL

Your partner lies on their side, leaning back a little, legs apart. You lie in front, backing onto the cock or dildo. Your thighs are together and resting between your partner's thighs. You can also get here by starting in Reverse Cowgirl, unbending your knees, and sending your legs out straight in front of you. And everyone tilts to the side.

TAKING THE L TRAIN

Your partner lies on their side. You lie on your side at a 90-degree angle— forming an L with your partner's body. Your chest faces the headboard. You bend your legs and put your knees over your partner's shoulders, your butt against the cock or dildo. Your partner enters you from there. Or try the above variation, where you're on your back.

Position:

STANDING

Description:

Standing face-to-face. It helps if you lift a leg and wrap it around your partner.

Pros:

- So sexy!
- Very intimate.
- Good for a quickie.

Cons:

- The thrusting is a little awkward.

Notes:

Nice against a wall for leverage and sexy fun times.

Standing Variations:

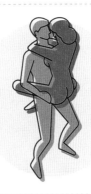

THE LIFTOFF

Your partner is standing and holds you by the butt as you straddle them. It takes a lot of strength. For greater ease and fun, your partner can hoist your butt on the kitchen counter (or washing machine or boss's desk).

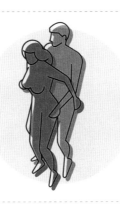

STANDING DOGGY

You stand and face away. Your partner enters you from behind. This position is tough if you are of different heights. (A possible solution? Sexy high heels on the shorter partner!) Or, you can get on all fours at the edge of the bed. Your partner stands and enters you from behind. Woof!

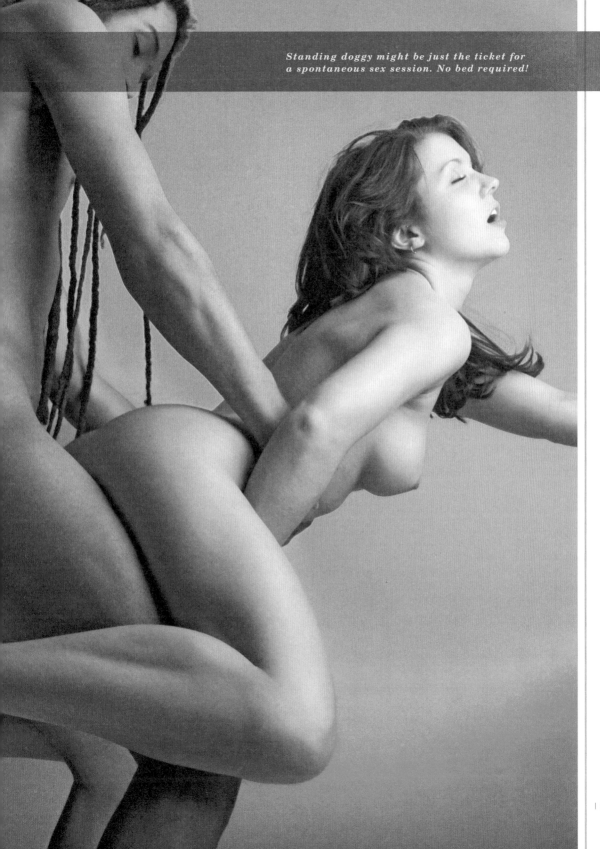

Position:

SITTING

Description:

Your partner sits in a chair–one without armrests. You sit and straddle your partner's lap in the chair. (Picture a Bob Fosse movie or a Madonna video.) You control all the action.

Pros:

- Nice and relaxing for your partner, who gets the ultimate lap dance and perfect breast access. And it's fun for you to have your partner at your command.
- You can control the exact depth of penetration.
- Good position for kissing and eye contact.

Cons:

- Your partner can't move very much.

Notes:

Everyone's hands are free for groping.
Your partner can help you with the work by grabbing your ass.

Sitting Variations:

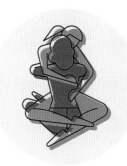

THE SWAMI

Your partner sits up in bed (legs out or cross-legged) and, facing each other, you sit on their lap, legs astride or around your partner. You can also transition to this from Cowgirl if your partner sits up and you straighten your legs. Great for closeness and kissing, since your chests come together in a hug. Arms are free. It takes some torso strength to stay upright.

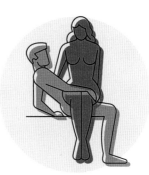

SIDESADDLE

This works well on an armchair. You sit on your partner's lap, but ride sidesaddle instead of astride. You move yourself up and down with your arms or your legs if they reach the floor.

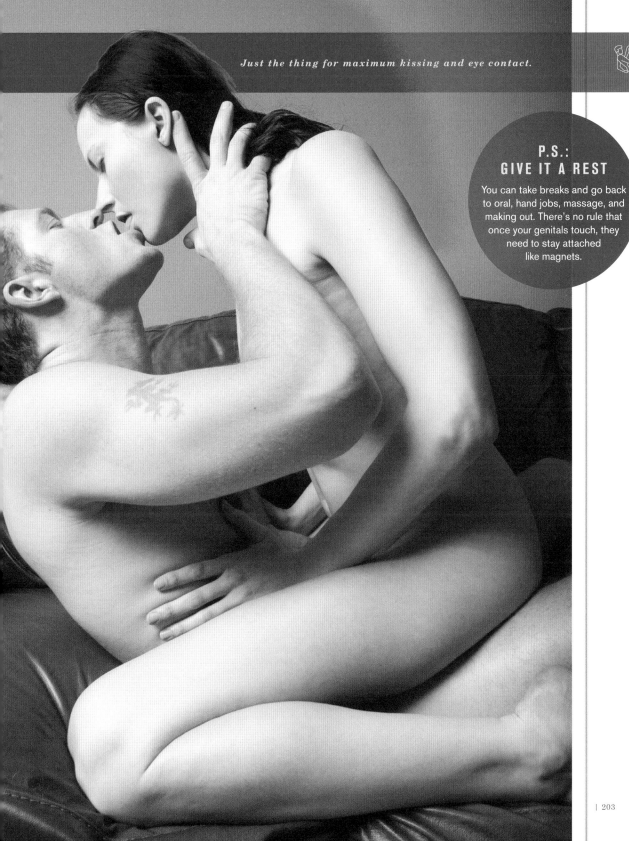

P.S.:
GIVE IT A REST

You can take breaks and go back to oral, hand jobs, massage, and making out. There's no rule that once your genitals touch, they need to stay attached like magnets.

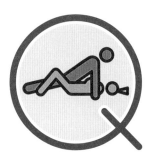

POSITION INQUISITIONS

{Q} "I really don't dig rear-entry positions. I feel like an animal, and I can't see anything. My partner really likes it though."

{A} For many, the animal feeling is a plus, but to each their own. If you miss the full-body contact of other positions, lying on your stomach and letting your partner lie on top of you, entering from behind, could feel better. If it's the view that makes you feel left out, try doing it doggy style in front of a mirror.

It can be thrilling to watch how excited your partner is to be moving inside you. If your cervix is getting bumped with a "feels too deep" sensation, ask for shallower thrusts and try curling your back up into a bridge. Alternatively, shallower thrusts plus an arched back may target your G-spot.

"I like being on top, but my man doesn't like it when I ride him."

{Q}

{A} First of all, make sure you aren't hurting him. Check to see that the angle is comfortable, and that you have enough lube for slippery slidey-ness. Keep as much weight as possible in your hands and knees so you don't squash his pelvis. We suspect that his cock feels OK, but his soul doesn't love being pinned down, unable to move. After, say, getting yelled at by his boss all day, it might not be fun to have his girlfriend ride him like a mule. So keep the power dynamic in mind and talk to him about how he feels. Spend some time in positions that give him control. Then it's just a matter of passing the reins back and forth. If Cowgirl is the best position (or only position) for you to come during intercourse, let him know—that should be powerful motivation for him to kick back and enjoy the ride.

"My boyfriend says I'm not tight enough. Can this be true?"

{Q}

{A} Nope. Your vagina isn't "too loose," any more than his penis is "too small." Your body is perfect just the way it is. This isn't a problem with your body—that he wants a tighter fit is something for you two to work on together. Remember, your vagina is two walls of muscle resting against each other. It's an envelope, not a tunnel. You can hold a tampon in there, so it's unlikely that you're too big for your man. Here are a few things to try: 1) You could do some Kegel exercises (see p. 23), which will strengthen the vaginal muscles so they hold more tension and you can even voluntarily clench around his penis—a nice move right before orgasm. 2) He can try putting a finger or two in you along with his cock. That might feel tighter for everybody. 3) Make sure to try some doggy style, which tends to feel tighter for the guy than face-to-face.

"Is it possible to orgasm without genital stimulation?"

{Q}

{A} We're big believers in whole-body sexuality. Sexual response isn't located in just our genitals. Bring in more parts of your body and you'll feel enlivened and can even have whole-body orgasms. If your clit or vulva is not responsive, you can still get off with stimulation to other parts of your body. People with different abilities, including people with spinal injuries, certain diseases, or other issues can enjoy a sexuality as robust as anyone's, including orgasm without genital involvement. Even if your clit is fully functional, it's great to expand your areas of exploration.

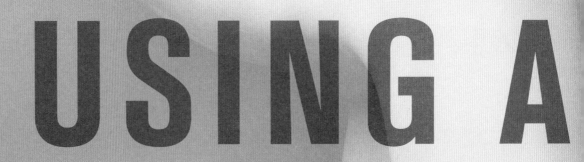

USING A

Some things to consider before strapping up: What kind of dildo does she like? How big? How realistic? You can get a dildo with balls, with veins—or something more sleek and sculptural. It definitely needs a flared base to keep it steady in the harness. We recommend a silicone toy (see The Satisfied Customer, p. 212).

STRAP-ON

You want vibration too? Get a vibrating dildo or add on a vibrating cock ring. Are you penetrating anally? Then you might want to start with something smaller than the average cock. How many fingers has your partner enjoyed up the bum? That's a good size indicator.

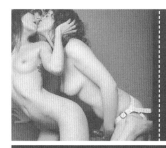
THE HARNESS

You've got options. Harnesses come in leather, rubber, spandex, and nylon webbing. The leather is extra sexy to many people. It warms and conforms to the body, but it can be pricier. Rubber and nylon are cheaper and easier to clean. There's the one-strap thong style and a two-strap jock style (which leaves your V available for fucking). Some have an extra pouch for tucking in a vibrator. Since a harness is a dramatic piece of sexual costumery, take a moment to savor your visual choices: masculine, feminine, SM-y, robot-y. Do you want to look like you just walked out of *The Matrix* or a bordello? (Both sound good to us!)

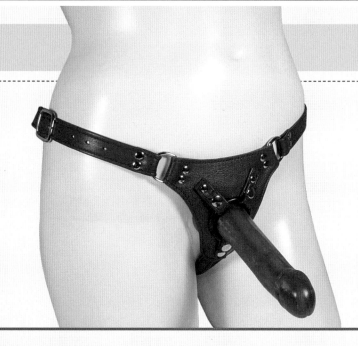

REHEARSING FOR YOUR BIG NIGHT

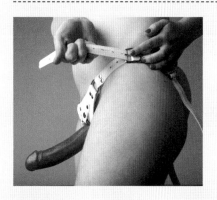

It's both wise and fun to play with your getup before you giddyap. This rehearsal will save you some awkwardness in the bedroom later. Place your dildo in the harness. Try the whole thing on and pull the straps tight. A tighter harness means a more solid and steady fit. You want to feel as connected as possible. Situate the dildo base higher up on the mons or smack dab over the clit. Most important, feel the connection to your body. Check your bad self out in the mirror. Hold your new cock and feel the zingy energy it gives you. Get connected to your "psychic dick." Maybe grab some lube and jerk it off for some real gender-bending fun. How does that feel? Take a picture with your phone and send it to your partner. (Just be sure it's addressed to "Dan" and not "Dad" before hitting send. Or maybe just keep the picture for yourself, to look at when life is boring.) In terms of prepping your partner, you've definitely penetrated them with fingers, right? If not, practice that way until you're both comfortable. (See p. 149.)

HOW TO START

1 Lube up and down the dildo's shaft.

2 Use your fingers to lube up your partner's orifice of choice. Rub and tease until he or she can't wait for what's next.

3 Replace your massaging fingers with the head of the dildo. Grasp the dildo's shaft so you can control the force and the depth. Gently push into the hole.

4 Start by only fucking the opening with the tip of your toy. As the pleasure builds, your partner's hips will rise to meet you and take in more.

5 Engage your core muscles, use your dirty talk, and let your partner know you love it!

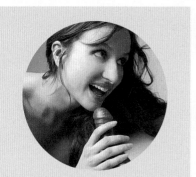

Don't forget you can have oral fun with a strap-on! See p. 179 for more details.

GALS FUCKING GUYS: PEGGING

Turnaround is fair play, people. For couples, it can be the ultimate act of empathy—each person is feeling the other's experience. Women can get a kick out of rocking a cock after years of being the cock receiver. And if a guy has been begging to give anal sex, a lady has every right to ask him to get it too. Everybody wins.

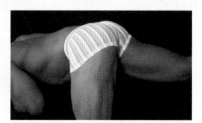

SEX TIPS FOR STRAPPERS

• You and your partner should decide together if you're going to fuck anally, vaginally, or both.

• Put a condom on beforehand if the dildo's going into more than one orifice.

• If you plan to go from butt to puss, just toss the condom after butt and before pussy—so simple!

• Get everyone's engines revved with manual and oral attentions. No need to go from zero-to-strap-on in sixty seconds.

• Unless you started out all suited up, you probably need to interrupt sex play to get into your gear. Let your partner help you get dressed to build anticipation (unless you want to run away and reappear becocked with a fabulous "Ta-da!").

• Get lots of feedback, especially if you are doing your partner anally. (See How to Start, at left.) Since you can't actually feel with your dildo, you might slip out.

• Keep watching your dildo work (why waste these visuals by fucking in the dark?) and hold your cock at the base if you need better connection and control. Before long it will feel like an extension of your body that you control with your hips and your mind.

• Keep the angle of your partner's butt or pussy in mind, especially if your dildo is pretty stiff. You have the luxury of turning your dildo upside-down if that helps. (Take that, human male!) Always try to angle it toward the belly, not the spine, so you are stimulating the prostate or G-spot. Enjoy!

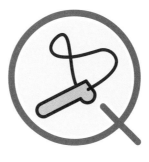

{ Q & A }

DILDO DILEMMAS

{Q} "I tried a strap-on and my girlfriend loved it, but how can I get more out of it for me?"

{A} The power and satisfaction of getting her off feels good and hopefully increases your own arousal. From that excited state, the energy and impact of the thrusting can give you enough stimulation to orgasm if the base of the dildo is in the right spot. You could also trick out the harness with a vibrator or use a vibrating cock, which will get your clit. A double-headed dildo may be the ticket. There's lots of stuff to try, so don't write it off too quickly.

{Q} "Why do we need toys? Shouldn't my partner be enough to get me off?"

{A} Well, you can have a fun day at the beach with just you, a friend, the sand, and the sea. But isn't the beach even more fun if you have a bucket, a shovel, a volleyball net, and a ball? Does that make you a beach cheater? We think bringing a sex toy to bed is like bringing a Frisbee to the beach: You can enjoy yourself without it, but why not play?

{Q} "What about dildos for couples?"

{A} Dildos that you've enjoyed for solo play are welcome in a twosome. You can put on a sultry sex show by using a dildo to masturbate for your partner, or by sucking it off with great verve—an act that says, "Yeah, that's right. I'm a badass sexpot." If you're curious about the joys of double penetration, try a dildo in your back door while your sweetheart fucks your front door (or the reverse). You get all the fun of a three-way without the potential hurt feelings. And, of course, you don't have to strap one on to enjoy dildos as a couple. Even watching your partner masturbate with one is still a shared sexual experience.

{Q} "What about double dildos? Do they really work?"

{A} Since we started selling toys, the double-head-ed dildo has evolved as a species. Now they are boomerang-shaped so that one end goes inside a woman (sort of like a butt plug for the pussy). A harness keeps that half in place, while she rocks the other dildo like a regular strap-on. She can penetrate a partner or even lube up and jerk it off—she'll feel the jerking internally instead of externally, which can be awesome.

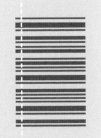

The
SATISFIED CUSTOMER

{THE DILDO GUIDE}

Dildo shopping involves a lot of personal preference. Shape, size, texture, style, and color are all up to you. We carry a large variety of dildos because everyone's desire is different. This quick guide is designed to hook you up with your dream dick. Plus, insights from our customers who have already taken one out for a spin.

"ARE THERE DILDOS THAT LOOK LIKE DICKS?"

If you're looking for a lifelike dildo, the Bandit is scandalously realistic. Made of medical-grade, velvety soft VixSkin silicone, and comes with a lifetime warranty.

What our customers say:

"My girlfriend and I have several toys, and the Bandit is by far our favorite! It fits in a harness perfectly, and it's realistic enough for any fantasy. I love to pack it too—it's perfect!"

"I CAN'T DEAL WITH A STRAP-ON."

Hand-held dildos like the Pure Wand are great for self-use and for folks who love penetration but don't want a strap-on.

What our customers say:

"Once you've tried the Pure Wand nothing else compares! It's hands down the best G-spot dildo ever! This toy goes everywhere my fingers cannot. The result? Only the best, most powerful orgasms of my life!"

"WE'D LOVE TO FIND SOMETHING WE CAN USE AT THE SAME TIME."

Double-ended dildos like the Share allow both partners to be penetrated simultaneously. Using a harness can make these dildos easier to control.

What our customers say:

"My girlfriend bought the Share for me as a gift, and I have to say it is the best toy I have ever had. The wearer's end gave me a blackout-inducing orgasm and the penetration end was super-fun to play with as well—both on me and on her."

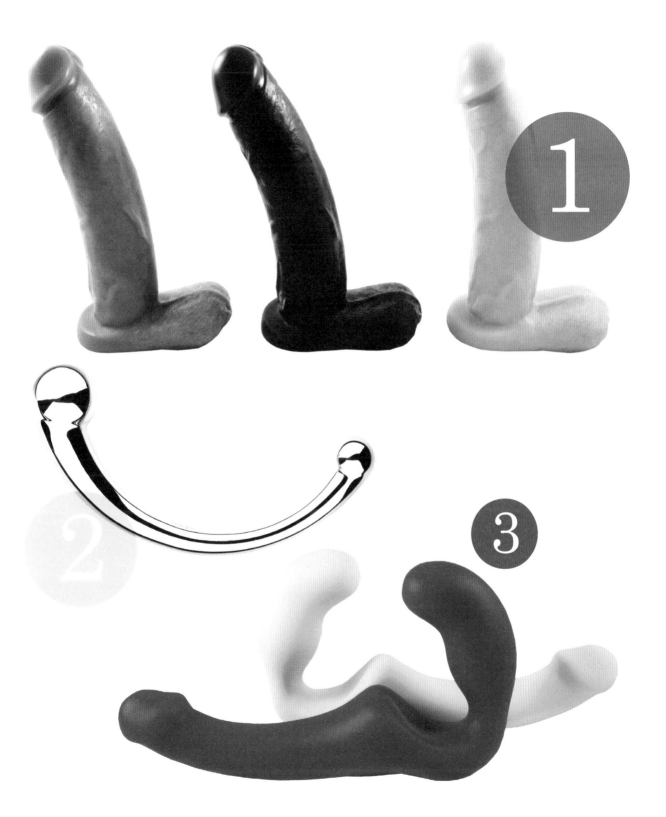

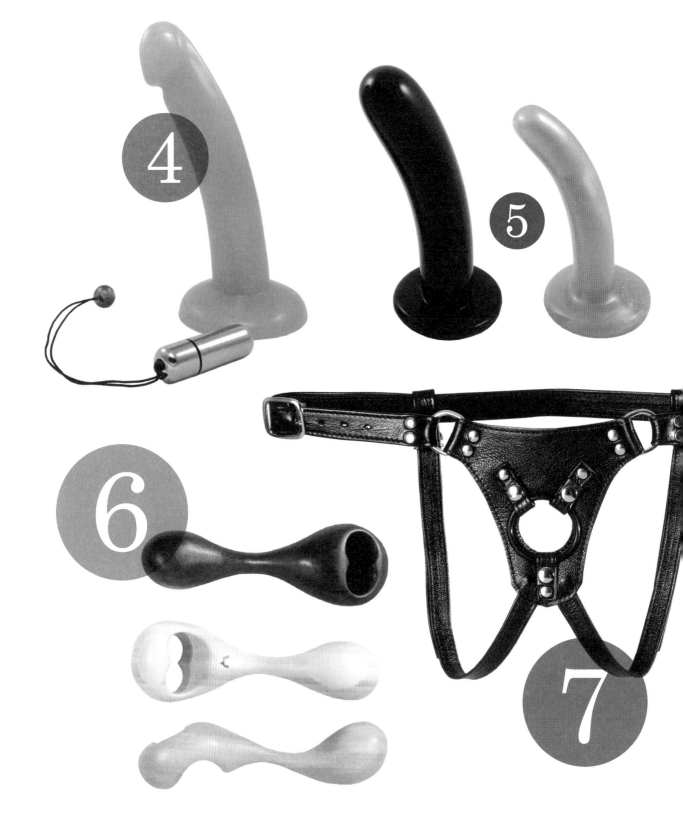

④ "IS THERE A TOY THAT CAN FILL ME UP–AND VIBRATE?"

The Vibrating Mistress is a silicone beauty that incorporates a mini-vibrator in the base. The vibrator can be removed during cleaning.

What our customers say:

"Wow, the Vibrating Mistress is just a fantastic dildo. It's a great size for backdoor play, and is nice and smooth and soft. The vibe just takes your breath away when you switch it on."

⑤ "I'D LIKE TO TRY PEGGING."

Smaller dildos like the Silk are great for anal-play beginners.

What our customers say:

"Guys! Don't knock it until you try it! One of my girlfriend's fantasies was to do me with a strap-on dildo in the butt. So she bought a harness and the small Silk for our first time. When she saw how intense my orgasm was, she had to give it a try!"

⑥ "IS THERE A DILDO THAT WILL HIT MY G-SPOT?"

Yup. G-spot toys all feature a distinct curve. If you're looking for targeted stimulation, try dildos with a curved tip, like the Fling.

What our customers say:

"Wow! The first thing that took me in was how sexy the sleek, organic shape of the Fling was. My partner and I love G-spot toys, but this one takes the cake! Unlike other G-spot toys, this one stays tucked against that sweet spot the whole time."

⑦ "I WANT A HARNESS FOR MY DILDO."

Easily the most beautiful and comfortable harness currently on the market is the Jaguar Harness. This ingenious design is made of soft and supple garment leather for easy wearing, and it fits like a glove!

What our customers say:

"This harness is great! It straps on easily and fits very comfortably once it's adjusted. It stays in place and the leather is very soft. I can wear it around the house without the strap digging into my skin. My girlfriend thinks it looks hot as well, and it holds large and small dildos wonderfully."

ANAL SEX:

THE BIG TABOO. The amount of tension surrounding anal sex might be directly proportionate to the amount of tension stored up in America's actual butt hole muscles. We've been taught since toddlerhood not to play with our assholes and to clench 'em tight when we feel sensation back

SPECIAL DELIVERY TO THE BACK DOOR

there. And we clench tighter and deeper when we are stressed, so no wonder it's tough to go to the back door for pleasure. And no wonder it's hard to think of the butt hole as sexy. But more and more people are finding that anal pleasure is amazing, and are inviting it to the big sex party.

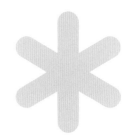

✳ THE ASS-VANTAGES

There are a ton of nerve endings around the anus—far more than there are around the vagina. As one of our Babeland sex educators is fond of saying, "If the vaginal opening had as many nerve endings as the anus, no woman in her right mind would give birth." All those nerves mean sensational possibilities for pure pleasure. Also, if you learn to work with your anal muscles, there are some medical advantages:

✳ You can release all that "tight-ass" tension.

✳ You can stimulate the muscles and tissue to help fight constipation and hemorrhoids.

✳ You'll get your sphincter muscles in top form, which will help prevent incontinence later. Rather than anal sex putting you in danger of needing adult diapers, done without force, it actually makes your bum healthier.

PAIN: THE MYTH AND THE REALITY

Anal sex shouldn't hurt or feel uncomfortable. If it does, stop and start over another way, or another day. People assume that anal sex is painful, but the fact is, if you're careful and patient, it shouldn't be. Some folks go a step further and think, "Oh, I just need to numb the pain so I/she/he can endure anal sex." There are creams on the market for this, and we hate them! Sex—anal and otherwise—should be felt and enjoyed, not numbed and endured. Furthermore, pain is the body's natural response to trauma, so numbing cream can, in some cases, stop you from knowing that something is wrong. One more thing on the pain tip: anal sex can give you new and unusual sensations. Sometimes a new or unusual feeling registers as pain because you're a little freaked out. Surprise! When you're exploring anal-land and something is alarming you, try and ask yourself (as you reach for the phone to dial 911), "Does this hurt or just feel weird?" If the answer is "It just feels weird," then keep going if you want to. Stop if it hurts.

SOLO PRACTICE

If pondering anal sex with a partner, consider trying it alone first. You can address your fears, find your boundaries, get comfortable with the sensations. Are you afraid you're going to poop all over yourself? (You won't, but fears are fears.) Then try it in the bathtub, where a mess is no biggie. You think it's dirty? Then put a glove or condom on your hand or toy for easy cleanup. Here's a helpful list of steps to follow if you're an anal-nooky newbie:

 Get your lube (since the butt hole is sensitive and makes no lube of its own) and get comfortable. If you're experimenting with a sex toy, make sure it has a flared base so you can always get it out.

 Try some garden-variety masturbation to get yourself in an erotic mood.

 Add some lube (if you didn't already), deep breathing, and anal massage to your self-love. Remember, once fingers go in the A-hole, they don't go back to the V-hole. Suggestion: Use two hands—one for frontsies, one for backsies. Do this until you feel relaxed and turned on.

 Bring the pad of the finger or top of a small sex toy to the anal opening, and rest it there while you inhale and bear down like you are trying to poop.

 Exhale and let the toy or finger slide in. If it hurts (not just feels weird, but hurts), back it out a little. Or stop altogether until you feel like trying again.

 If an object goes into your rectum but seems to "hit a wall" about four inches in, then pull the toy gently out and try angling it up toward your belly. You have to respect and follow the curve of the rectum (see Your Butt, p. 26).

 Wiggle, slowly thrust, or otherwise play until you've had enough.

 Call your boss, mom, or congressional representative to tell them about your latest adventure! (Kidding.)

HAVE BUTT-ASS-TIC SEX WITH YOUR PARTNER

BRING YOUR LUBE AND YOUR NEWFOUND KNOWLEDGE INTO THE BEDROOM.

Demonstrate the steps on the previous page, either on yourself (sexy show-and-tell!) or on your partner. Or show your partner how to do the steps to you—with finger, toy, or penis. As with the solo version, you two don't have to tackle all the steps in one session. Just play until you've had enough. Try warming up with a rim job (oral to anal—see Rim Job Recipe, p. 166). If you're getting close to orgasm right before moving on to anal sex, you can try stopping before you come. Or you can go ahead and have your first orgasm, which leaves you relaxed and loosey-goosey. Either is good. If one of you is anally fucking the other, remember the

Babeland ass rules: relax and go slowly (and avoid the wild thrusting—leave that to the porn stars), communicate ("Not yet, sailor—but I liked the massage"), and lube it up like you've got stock in the product. Once you're in, try to angle the penis or toy to stimulate the G-spot through the vaginal wall, or the prostate in a man. Both are about two inches in and toward the belly side.

Once you're comfortable, you and your partner can experiment with some of the positions on the facing page.

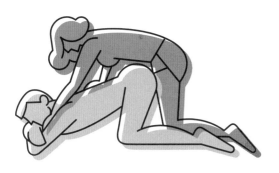

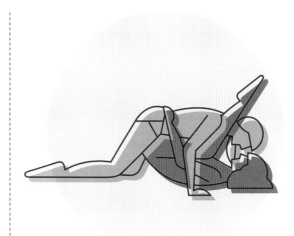

DOGGY STYLE

The penetrate-ee (bottom) can have their torso upright (like kneeling in prayer) or across (on all fours) or down (chest on bed). The bottom has some control over depth and angle of penetration. The top has a great view and a lot of control.

MISSIONARY

The bottom person's legs are in the air, presenting the butt hole to the sky (and partner). The top person controls the movement and penetration, but the bottom person has decent control over the angle.

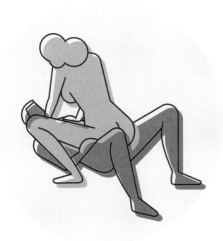

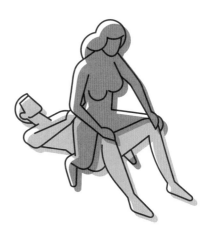

COWGIRL/COWBOY

One person straddles the penetrator and inserts the dildo or penis anally ("Like sitting on a fencepost," one customer said). While the cowpoke is getting poked, they can control the angle and the movement. Good for eye contact.

REVERSE COWGIRL/COWBOY

Same as at left, but facing away, which might be a better angle for penetration. (Not as good for eye contact, obviously.)

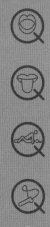

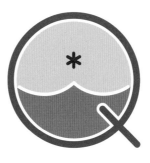

ANAL ASKS

{Q} ## "I'm afraid to get poo on me. Totally ew."

{A} Yes, you poop out of your anus. Then the poop goes in the toilet and the rectum is empty, with perhaps some traces of poop on the rectum walls. Future poop is higher up in the intestine, out of reach of fingers and dildos and penises. As long as your partner recently emptied out their rectum (which is the polite thing to do), you are not going to prod into their back alley and feel a big turd. Every anal-sex receiver is the best judge of whether it's a good day to have anal sex or not. Communicating about that will help avoid any major encounters with poop. You might encounter tiny traces from the rectal walls,

which are harmless to your fingers. Just don't let those fingers visit a vagina without a good washing, because the butt bacteria can cause a urinary tract infection or BV. You can wear a rubber finger cot (available in pharmacies) or glove if you want to stay squeaky clean during anal expeditions. A penis going into a butt hole should wear a condom so it doesn't pass on any STIs. If going to the vagina from the ass, dildos, fingers, penises, or anything else should wear a barrier that you can whisk off. If not, pause to wash up. You can also perform an anal douche an hour or so beforehand if you really want to be uber-clean for inspection (water or saline only!). But it's not necessary.

"Does any woman enjoy anal sex the way guys dig it?"

Hells, yeah! But let's just say that more men come into the shop and ask, "How do I get my girl to do anal?" than women trying to get their guys to do it to them. In fact, a lot of women come in and ask, "My boyfriend really wants to have anal sex—can you help me?" So by that unscientific survey, we'd say more guys want this. That might also be true because: 1) Guys like to stick their dicks somewhere tight, and the butt is generally tighter than the vagina. And 2) In traditional man/woman anal sex, it's the woman who is vulnerable and feels like she could get hurt. That might keep the female number down. But plenty of women love it, and many hetero couples do it at least sometimes. We also get men who ask us how to convince their lovers to peg them. As knowledge replaces phobias, the balance is shifting to a more equal place.

"Is there any difference between a man receiving anal penetration and a woman receiving anal penetration?"

Anatomically speaking, yes, but not enough to justify the hype about it. Men have a prostate gland ("the male G-spot") that is reachable through the rectum, about two inches inside the anus, toward the belly. Anal sex and anal play can give guys mind-bending pleasure because the prostate positively adores the attention. But don't be too envious, ladies. The wall between the rectum and the vagina is quite thin, and a toy or penis up the female bum can stimulate your G-spot though the wall if it's angled toward the belly just right. Women also have the option of double penetration—a penis/toy/finger in both the vagina and the anus.

"My boyfriend loves receiving anal sex. Is he gay?"

No. He's with you, right? Desire for other men might mean he's bi, but that's about desire, not butt-fucking. Your boyfriend has discovered his prostate. He's found more ways to enjoy his body. And the better he is at finding pleasure, the better he probably is at giving it. You've got a secure and sensual man on your hands.

The
SATISFIED
CUSTOMER

{THE ANAL GUIDE}

Plugs! Beads! Dildos! There are loads of ways to enjoy anal sex. And for everything you might want to do, there's a toy to help you do it. Butt plugs, anal beads, and smooth, slim dildos each stimulate the ass in their own specific way. Here's a guide to help you fulfill your butt-sex dreams.

"I'M A COMPLETE BEGINNER AT THIS. WHAT'S A GOOD FIRST PLUG?"

Try our smallest plugs, the Little Flirt and Bootie. Both are easy-to-clean silicone and small enough to help a novice ease into the wonderful world of butt sex. Their tiny size makes each great for the first outing, but they may need a little help staying in.

What our customers say:

"The right position or garment will hold it in. I have used all manner of sex toys, and it is still my all-time favorite! It definitely provides an amazing climax; don't underestimate the Little Flirt. It's a little treasure!"

"As a couple beginning to explore anal play, we have found the Bootie to be a sensational toy, especially for beginners who may want to prepare for strap-on play like us. We recently discovered that if I rub my vibrator over the part of the Bootie that is flush against his ass, the vibrations get carried through the Bootie and drive him wild. He feels he can almost orgasm without even touching his cock!"

"WHAT ARE BUTT BEADS? WHICH SHOULD I TRY?"

Butt beads are series of knobs or balls that graduate in size, attached along a string or a flexible stalk. They make the anus open and close over and over as they go in, and, delightfully, as you pull them out, preferably during orgasm. Flexi Felix is a great example of this design. The Ripple has the undulating shape of butt beads, but also has the classic flared base of a butt plug.

What our customers say:

"I had always been a little wary of butt play, but the Flexi Felix looked so cute I just couldn't resist buying it. It's soft and flexible, unlike other beads I looked at and the shape of the beads makes them easy to insert and remove."

"The Ripples are my first experience with anal play. I'm having an unbelievable experience, especially when I added a massager for vibrations. With just a little patience it slides in beautifully and gives a nice feeling of fullness."

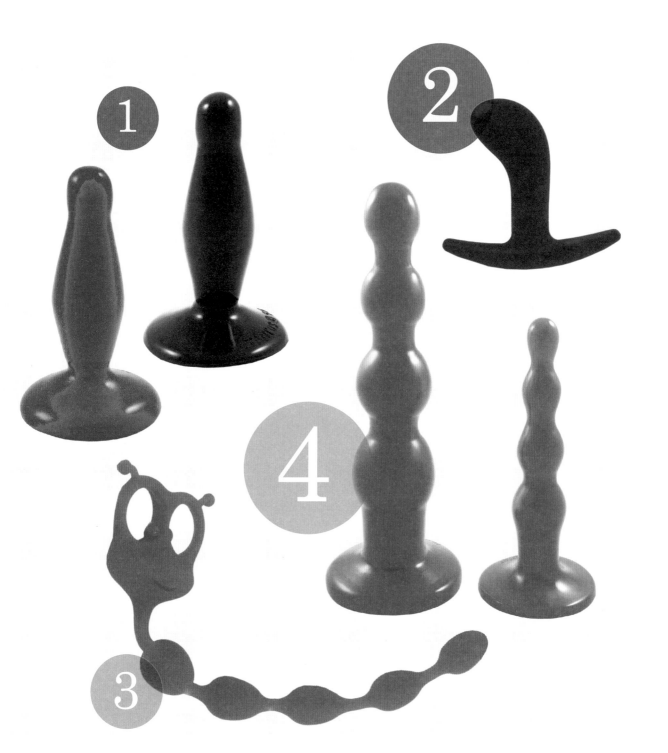

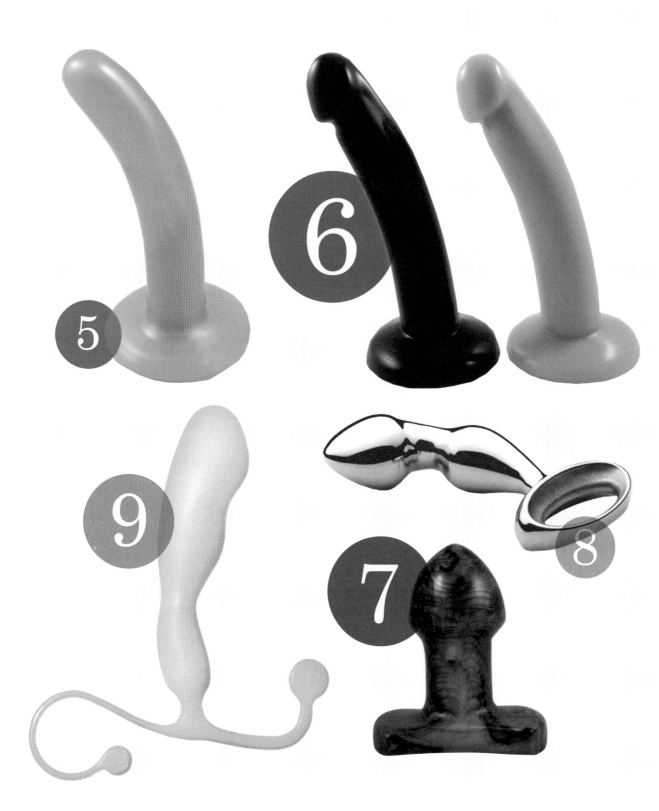

"I WANT A DILDO FOR ANAL PLAY."

Almost any dildo will do for anal play. That said, a lot of folks prefer a smooth dildo that's not too big around. The Silk line of dildos is ideal for smooth, easy in-and-out penetration. Silk comes in a variety of lengths and widths, and has no challenging curves or bumps. Mistress, another great choice, is a tapering, slender toy with a hint of a head on the tip, that comes with or without a vibrator inside.

What our customers say:

"My girlfriend and I are new to anal toys. Tried our first today and weren't disappointed! This cute little pink guy works well as a plug (stayed put during sex) or for in-and-out motion. Highly recommend Silk for anal beginners."

"The Mistress worked great for my girlfriend, who doesn't like too much girth. It worked great for my boyfriend, who loved the curve and slender shaft. It worked great for me because it looked super-sexy in my harness."

"I WANT A PLUG THAT WILL STAY WHERE I PUT IT, HANDS-FREE."

Medium-size plugs with a thin waist (for your sphincter to close around) that leads to a flared base are your best bet for staying in. You may need to train your body to hold on to any toy during the throes of orgasm. The Tristan has a bulbous head, a thin waist, and little scoops cut out of the base for butt-cheek comfort.

What our customers say:

"The Tristan is my first good-size butt plug. I just love the fabulous stretch putting it in. I like to go nice and slow and feel the plug going in ever so slowly. Once it's in, a good strong vibrator applied to the base is magnificent. I'm coming all over the place in no time."

"MY BOYFRIEND WANTS TO TRY A PROSTATE MASSAGE."

Guys are realizing more and more that their butts are the gateway to a new, incredibly satisfying realm of sexual pleasure. The Aneros prostate stimulator and the Pfun Plug each offer the angle and firmness needed to give his prostate a thrill ride.

What our customers say:

"The Pfun is the best thing I've ever stuck in my butt, and I have a drawer full of toys to compare it with. It can really send me into orbit with minimal additional physical or mental stimulation. My girl likes it in her ass or pussy too, for the weight and bumpy-ness."

"Aneros is not hype. It requires practice and time to get the hang of it. Once mastered, you won't believe your body was capable of generating so much pleasure! I had an orgasm that lasted three hours. It kept building and building."

CHAPTER 7

A LIFETIME OF GOOD SEX:

SAFER, HOTTER, *and* BETTER

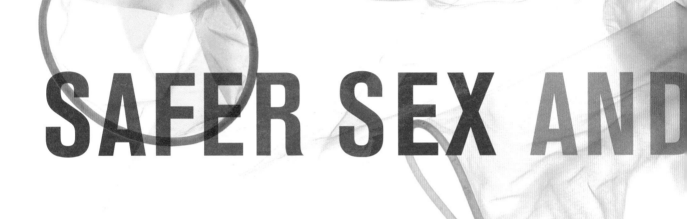

SAFER SEX AND

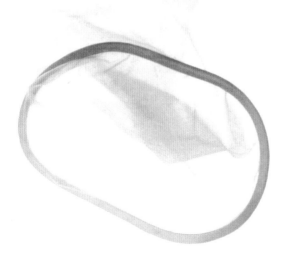

BIRTH CONTROL

Here are the basics, and some questions you might want to ask yourself (and your doctor). All the latex in the world won't do you any good unless you plan ahead, use your smarts, and communicate with your partner. The good news is that safer sex doesn't have to be a drag. We think condoms and gloves and dams and lube are fun to play with—bright colors, all kinds of textures and sensations. And that's the key:

WORK SAFER SEX INTO YOUR NAKED PLAYTIME

and soon enough it's a habit that just feels normal and good, like brushing your teeth.

THE OTHER SAFER SEX

Safer sex generally means using latex or other non-porous barrier methods to prevent fluid contact during sexual activities. But let's not forget that there are all kinds of ways to get off with little or no risk of catching a bug: massage, hand jobs, dry humping, mutual masturbation, vibe and dildo play, making out, fantasizing, phone sex, sexting, and so on. (See the rest of this book!) You might think, "Oh, I'm a grown-up now. Grown-ups have sex. I left dry humping behind in tenth grade." But remember how much fun that all was in tenth grade? If you haven't had The Talk or you don't feel ready to deal with safe-sex issues or risks, then just take it slow. There's plenty you can do and enjoy.

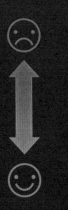

WHY IT'S CALLED "SAFER SEX":
ASSESSING RISK

It's called safer sex because you can't guarantee 100 percent risk-free sex. It's just like you can't guarantee a 100 percent risk-free car ride, so you buckle up and drive safely, knowing that's the best you can do. Sexual activities range from a high degree of risk (bareback anal sex) to very low risk (kissing, massage). Some STIs (herpes, genital warts, or HPV) can be transmitted through skin contact. Others travel through blood and semen. Vaginal fluids are less likely to carry infection, and if they do it's probably in smaller doses. Saliva is a low-risk fluid. Here's a rough list of risks from high to low to help you assess:

HIGH RISK	• Anal sex without a condom • Vaginal sex without a condom • Oral sex on a menstruating woman
POSSIBLY RISKY	• Rim job (oral on anal) without a barrier • Blow job with swallowing • Sharing sex toys without using condoms or cleaning between uses • Cunnilingus without a barrier
LESS RISKY	• Blow job without swallowing • Manual sex (anal or vaginal) without a barrier
EVEN LESS RISKY	• Blow job with a condom • Cunnilingus with a barrier
SAFER	• Finger-fucking (anal or vaginal) with a barrier • Sharing sex toys, if using condom or cleaning between uses
EVEN SAFER	• Kissing

WHEN IS IT OK TO STOP USING PROTECTION?

Sorry, but people lie. People get embarrassed. Or some folks just bury their heads in the sand of ignorance and assume everything is fine. ("Oh, yeah, I'm totally STI-free. I think. Yeah—er, uh—totally.") Many people carry an STI and have no idea. If you aren't sure of the health status of a partner, protect yourself until you are. Or you can just take matters in your own hands and say, "Hey, let's get tested together" or "I'll go with you to get your checkup if you'll go with me to mine."

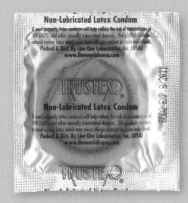

CONDOM-O-RAMA CHOICES!

Once you embrace the condom as your barrier method of choice, you have even more options.

SIZES, TEXTURES, AND FLAVAS

There are different sizes—from large to extra snug. There are condoms with cleverly designed room at the top, which allows more sensation for the penis. Check out the Inspiral to see how a soft-serve-inspired tip can make a big difference in the feel. There are condoms with texture either inside or outside, condoms with or without lubricant, and flavored condoms (nice for BJs!). If you are sensitive or allergic to latex, you can get condoms made of polyurethane—it's nice and thin but less stretchy, so more vulnerable to breakage. There's also a new material called polyisoprene that is a thin and stretchy alternative to latex. We recommend trying a bunch of types to see which one works for you and your partner.

FOR PROBLEMS WITH LATEX

If you think you have a sensitivity or allergy to latex condoms, the problem might be with the added "bonus" lubricant that's on 'em. So before you give up on latex, buy some unlubed latex condoms. Then, when you're in the moment, add some high-quality water-based lube. Lube prevents the condom from breaking and feels good.

If you or your partner still find the latex irritating, then move on to polyurethane or polyisoprene with greater clarity about the source of the problem. (Thank you, science.)

THE FEMALE CONDOM

Maybe it sounds like a contradiction in terms but, yes, there's a female condom. And, yes, men can use it too. It's actually quite popular in Europe, but the female condom hasn't really caught on stateside. You can get them in some drugstores and most sex-toy shops (see our Web site). What's great about the female condom? It empowers anyone on the receiving end to take charge and control safe sex. So if a guy is all, "My little guy doesn't want a raincoat on," then you can say, "OK. I'll wear the gear, dear." It's shaped like a large condom and has two flexible rings: a bigger one at the opening and a smaller one at the tip of the pouch. You pinch shut the smaller ring and insert it into your vagina much like you would a diaphragm, or remove the smaller inner ring and wear it in your anus. The larger ring stays outside the vagina or anus—a nice bonus is that it covers the labia and nearby ass skin so you get extra skin protection. The female condom is made of polyurethane, the less stretchy stuff, so use plenty of lube and don't play too rough, either.

CONDOM *and* DENTAL DAM DOs

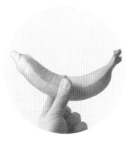

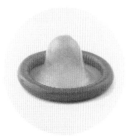

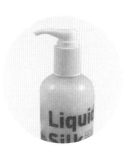

CONDOMS:

• DO practice putting a condom on a banana if you're a newbie.

• DO make sure you can tell the right side from the wrong side. If you have the right side up, the ring of rubber unrolls easily.

• DO add a drop of lube (just a dab!) to the inside tip–for his pleasure, and to minimize friction, which can cause condoms to break.

• DO pinch and hold the receptacle tip with your fingers or mouth when you unroll. This leaves room for the semen. Unroll all the way.

• DO have him hold the condom at the base when he pulls out so it doesn't stay inside the vagina or anus.

DENTAL DAMS:

• DO rinse off your dental dam if it has a fine powder on it.

• DO mark one side so that you know which side is up in case it slips.

• DO put a dab of lube on the lickee's side for extra goodness, if you like.

• DO use nonporous plastic wrap instead of a dam if you are in a pinch. You can also cut open a condom or latex glove and lay it flat.

CONDOM *and* DENTAL DAM DON'Ts

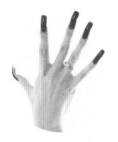

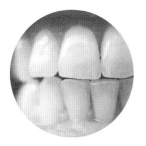

CONDOMS:

- DON'T open the package with your teeth or sharp nails, lest you cut or tear the condom, rendering it useless.

- DON'T use a condom that's past the expiration date, brittle, or gummy.

- DON'T store condoms near a source of heat. This can degrade the latex.

- DON'T double-bag. It can seem like two condoms are better than one, but they will rub against each other and could break.

DENTAL DAMS:

- DON'T reuse condoms or dams. Like they sing in Dreamgirls, these latex lovelies are for "One Night Only"!

- DON'T let it drop while in use. Licker should hold it in place. (Lickee can help during pussy licking. Tougher to do if you are using it anally.)

SEXUALLY TRANSMITTED INFECTIONS:
THE A-LIST

HIV/AIDS

HIV stands for human immunodeficiency virus, the virus that causes AIDS. (AIDS stands for acquired immunodeficiency syndrome.) The "immunodeficiency" part means that the disease breaks down the immune system, allowing infections and diseases (ones the body can normally fight off) to take over. The "acquired" part means people get it from infected blood, semen, or vaginal fluid that has reached their mucous membranes or open cuts somewhere. HIV is most commonly spread through unprotected vaginal or anal sex, or through needle sharing. Latex, along with open and honest communication, is your best friend when it comes to HIV prevention.

HERPES

Herpes is a virus that causes painful sores (outbreaks). The first outbreak is the worst. The rest can usually be suppressed with antiviral drugs, but stress or other illnesses can trigger an outbreak. There are many strains of herpes. A cold sore on your mouth typically signifies a less severe form of herpes. Important: DO NOT perform oral sex if you have a cold sore, because you can turn your oral herpes into someone else's genital herpes. There's no cure for this STI.

HPV (GENITAL WARTS)

HPV stands for human papillomavirus, which causes genital warts. HPV is transmitted from skin-to-skin contact. There are almost one hundred strains of this virus, about twenty of which can affect the genitals. The warts are often too small to see with the naked eye, so you can't judge someone's health by sight. Sometimes the warts get bigger and nubbier and need to be burned or frozen off—a procedure well worth preventing. HPV can affect cell growth and cause some kinds of cervical and anal cancers. Pap smears test for unusual cervical cell growth caused by HPV, and anal pap smears are becoming more common (for both men and women). As we write, there is one vaccine available for young women ages ten to twenty-six that decreases the transmission of some of the most dangerous HPV strains. If you're within this age range, it's worth discussing the vaccine with your doctor, as HPV is widespread.

CHLAMYDIA

This is one of the most common STIs in the country. That's because the majority of people who have it show no symptoms, so these folks remain oblivious and keep passing it on through unprotected sexual contact. Chlamydia can be diagnosed through a simple urine test. It is super easy to treat with antibiotics, but be sure to retest for it a few months later, as the rate of reinfection is high. If left untreated, chlamydia can cause a more serious infection in women that can affect fertility later.

BUT WAIT, THERE'S MORE . . .

There are many other STIs out there, but if you're practicing safer sex, you're protecting yourself from these, too. Hepatitis B is a virus that affects the liver, and you can get a vaccine to prevent it. Gonorrhea and syphilis sound like mythical monsters, but they are very real (and treatable) bacterial infections. These two often show no symptoms but can damage your body if untreated over time, so get tested. Pubic lice (crabs) and scabies are tiny critters that live on skin, feed on blood, and spread from person to person. Though they spread through sexual contact, you can also get them from shared bedsheets, towels, or clothes. Both bugs are small and fairly difficult to see with the naked eye, so a doctor should diagnose you. Treatments are straightforward, and effective shampoos and creams are available. If you or a partner have itchy symptoms, get checked and then wash everything in super hot water. Housemates and family members should check for symptoms too. Bottom line: safer sex protects you from much more than HIV. If you ever have painful urination, severe itching, vaginal or penile discharge, or pain during sex, see your doctor, as these could be symptoms of an STI.

LIVING WITH AN ONGOING STI: HIV AND HERPES

No one with an STI needs to walk around in shame. If you've tested positive for an STI, you now have to be mature, smart, and communicative in your sexual encounters—that's a good thing. And you certainly don't have to tell anyone about your HIV or herpes unless it is the doctor treating you or a person interested in hooking up with you. Speaking of sex, there are dating sites and organizations just for people with HIV or herpes. These are places where you can skip the anxiety of The Big Talk and the stigma that often accompanies discussion of STIs and find people who know what it's like. If you're living with a virus, take meds as directed and help your body out with healthy living—good diet, exercise, and no harmful recreational drugs. It's what we all should do anyway.

BIRTH CONTROL:

MAKING CHOICES

Every time you have man/woman vaginal sex, there's a chance you could become pregnant. Like politicians love to tell us, abstinence is the only 100 percent effective method of birth control. How realistic is that for living as a sexual being? Not very. Since you're probably having sex or planning to, let's look at the most common methods out there.

BIRTH CONTROL PILLS

Birth control pills (a.k.a. the Pill) have a 92 to 98 percent effectiveness rate, which is pretty damn good. When used correctly—following medication instructions and not skipping pills—the Pill's failure rate drops to less than 1 percent. If you're on the Pill and use condoms, then you're fairly well protected from STIs and unwanted pregnancy (as the Pill does not protect against STIs). The Pill, which you take every day (no exceptions), delivers a low dose of hormone that prevents a woman from ovulating. No egg, no pregnancy. Then you stop taking the Pill or take placebos for one week, allowing you to menstruate. When you're on the Pill, your period is lighter, with less-severe cramps. (Some women take it just for that reason.) But there are sometimes undesirable side effects: breast tenderness, bloating, weight gain, moodiness, nausea. These symptoms may go away after a month or two. There are more serious risks if you are a smoker, are over thirty-five, or have diabetes or high cholesterol. This is something to discuss with your doctor.

OTHER HORMONAL METHODS

The birth control vaginal ring, the birth control patch, the birth control implant, and the birth control shot all work much like the Pill does, but they deliver hormones in other ways. The vaginal ring encircles your cervix and dissolves small amounts of hormone that get absorbed through the vaginal walls. The implant is a matchstick-size piece of plastic inserted under the skin of the upper arm, the patch sends the drug though your skin, and the shot is an injection. These carry similar risks, side effects, and benefits as the Pill. If you have trouble keeping track of your pill, consider one of these.

CONDOMS

Condoms are only about 75 to 85 percent effective over the long haul, which isn't great. If you are extra careful about using them right (rolling them on and off correctly, not breaking them, using lube), your chances can get a little better. But hey, it only takes one mess-up to get pregnant. We recommend combining condoms with another birth control method, like the

Pill. As for spermicide, some condoms come with spermicide, some people add spermicide, and the diaphragm method requires spermicide. A formerly popular one called nonoxynol-9 is getting phased out of the marketplace because it's extremely harsh on vaginal and anal tissue, and even causes little abrasions that make you more vulnerable to infection. Make sure you aren't using condoms with nonoxynol-9. Even other spermicides can be irritating and can throw off the pH balance of your vaginal juices, the body's natural cleansing system, leading to infection. We're not big fans.

IUD

That stands for intra-uterine device, and it's making quite a comeback. It's 99 percent effective—as effective as a vasectomy, except it's easily reversible. You just get it removed, and you're back in the fertility business. The IUD is cost-effective, too. After the initial insertion, it works for five to twelve years. So what is it, exactly? It's a small T-shaped device that your doctor inserts into your uterus via your cervix. Some are made of copper and others are plastic, containing hormones that dissolve slowly. Truth be told, doctors still aren't sure exactly how or why it prevents pregnancy, but it does something to the uterus or uterine lining that either sperm or fertilized eggs don't like. In the '70s and '80s, IUDs became unpopular due to a high rate of infections. But since then, medical folks have improved them, and IUDs have developed a good safety record.

DIAPHRAGMS AND THE SPONGE

Both of these work in a similar way, and both are about as effective as condoms for birth control—that is, not bad, not great. The diaphragm is a flexible rubber disc. You add spermicidal jelly to the center and edges, fold it like a taco, and insert it vaginally, covering the cervix like a dome. (Your ob-gyn can help you practice.) The sponge is available in drugstores—which is nice—and

has the spermicide built in. You wet it and insert it much the same way you do the diaphragm. Yes, these both put the woman in control: you can insert either of these discs hours before sex. But the spermicide can be abrasive and messy. We're not huge fans.

EMERGENCY CONTRACEPTION

It's also called the Morning After Pill, or goes by the brand name Plan B. If a condom breaks, or you have a birth control snafu, or you had sex you didn't want (possibly rape, in which case you should seek counseling), emergency contraception gives you another chance to prevent pregnancy. You can take emergency contraception up to five days after unprotected sex—but the sooner you do, the more effective it'll be. Pregnancy doesn't begin until a) the egg is fertilized, and b) the fertilized egg implants in the uterine wall. These steps take a few days, so emergency contraception intervenes before the pregnancy begins. The Morning After Pill does *not* cause an abortion. It's a high dose of hormone that prevents ovulation and makes the uterine lining unwelcoming to a fertilized egg. It's not one pill, as the name "Morning After Pill" would imply. It's a group of pills you take in one or two batches. They might make you feel nauseated, and if you throw them up, you have to start over. If you are sexually active, you might want to ask your doctor to prescribe emergency contraception so you can go get it if you ever need it. DO NOT just raid your roommate's birth control pills. Emergency contraception is a specific dosage that your doc should supervise.

TRACKING YOUR CYCLE, PULLING OUT

These are not reliable methods of birth control. Do we need to explain why? You can ovulate at almost any time and/or be fooled into thinking that mid-month bleeding is your period. As for pulling out, there's some sperm in the pre-come before then, and it just takes one little swimmer to fertilize an egg.

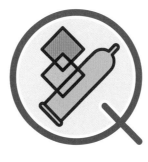

{ Q & A }

SAFER-SEX Qs

{Q} "At what point do you need to have 'the talk' about protection with a new partner?"

{A} Talk or no talk, safer sex is a commitment you make to yourself. Having your own set of rules—"I don't have sex unless there's a condom"—will make it about you, not the other person. And when you're fooling around, all hot and heavy, and clothes are coming off, that is a bad time to have a safer-sex discussion. Blood has traveled from your brain to your pants and judgment is cloudy. If you have made it to that point without discussion, we hope you'll have the wherewithal to stick to your rules and grab a condom or dam. Chatting sooner—when you're at dinner, say, or taking a walk—is a good idea. The conversation might take place sometime after you've made out a couple of times and you're pretty certain sex is in your future. Here are some things you might say:

• "I'm so excited about our date Thursday. I can't wait to see you naked. I've been tested for stuff, but I still use condoms. You cool with that?"

• "I'm hitting the drugstore tomorrow—you have a condom brand you like?"

• "No glove, no love."

Feel free to giggle and acknowledge any awkwardness. Your partner will probably be relieved that you brought it up first. If you know you have an STI, you absolutely must bring it up before the boots start knockin'. This can be tough, but it is your responsibility to tell a partner so he or she can make an informed decision about moving forward. (See Living With an Ongoing STI, p. 237.)

"How do I incorporate safer sex into sex play?"

{Q}

{A} Don't make getting a condom, dam, or glove a big interruption. Have it nearby, like any sex toy, and just work it into the game. Don't wait for your partner to go get the condom/dam/glove—let it be your job. Also have your lube nearby. Taking responsibility for your health is empowering and puts that one worry out of your mind so you can lose yourself safely in the sex. Once the condom is on the cock, or the dam is on the vag, you don't have to dive right into the main course. Maintain the sexual charge even after you bring out the latex. Just like waiting for your food in a restaurant, sex always tastes better after you've been craving it longer. For a great party trick, see p. 160 for how to put on a condom with your mouth.

"I just don't use condoms for giving blow jobs and am not sure I ever will. Am I doomed?"

{Q}

{A} Not necessarily. Just be aware of the risk you are accepting. You greatly reduce the dangers if you don't swallow any semen. It's possible (though pretty rare) to get gonorrhea or chlamydia in your throat. Does your partner have herpes or HPV? Those can be passed on from skin-to-skin contact even if you do use a condom. (There could be a sore or warts on his balls or another area the condom doesn't cover.) If you are longtime monogamous partners with up-to-date doc visits, your risk is pretty low. IMPORTANT TIP: don't give head (and especially don't let him come in your mouth) soon after you've flossed or brushed your teeth. Flossing and brushing cause lots of tiny little abrasions that are vulnerable to germs and infection.

"Can a person have sex after getting HIV?"

{Q}

{A} Yes, but someone with HIV or AIDS must inform partners. And, of course, safer sex is a must to prevent possible contact with blood, semen, or vaginal fluid (saliva, tears, sweat, and urine aren't dangerous). Since AIDS was recognized in the early '80s, medicine has made huge advances, and people with HIV and AIDS are living totally normal lives for much longer. There are combinations of meds (a.k.a. "cocktails") that suppress the virus. This is great news for happy living, but we hope it doesn't make people complacent about safer sex: "Oh, they've got AIDS under control now" or "Hey, he looks healthy to me so there can't be a dangerous infection in the picture." Don't be misled—HIV and AIDS are serious business, and there is still no known cure.

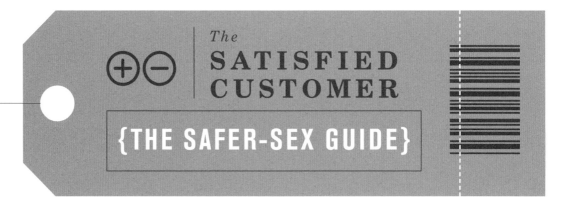

The
SATISFIED CUSTOMER

{THE SAFER-SEX GUIDE}

"I LIKE A LUBED-UP CONDOM. WHADDYA GOT?"

Try the Babeland Condom, thin, silky-smooth latex that transmits body heat beautifully between partners, allowing maximum sensation for the wearer. Plus, it's pre-lubed to keep things gliding along. Basic, versatile, smooth, and strong—we like our condoms like that, and we think you will too.

What our customers say:

"This is one amazing condom. In addition to making things feel more natural to me, my girlfriend was convinced that my dick was bigger. There really isn't any more I can say."

"MY GIRLFRIEND IS ALLERGIC TO LATEX, SO I NEED A GOOD ALTERNATIVE."

Lifestyles Skyn condoms are a new alternative to latex condoms that doesn't sacrifice body heat and closeness. They're made of polyisoprene, a natural rubber with the strength and sensitivity of latex. And they're even thinner than most latex condoms. Avoid oil-based lubes with use.

What our customers say:

"I love these! I'm mildly allergic to latex—which didn't occur to me until after I tried these and I no longer was sore after sex. They feel ten times better than latex— and have no taste whatsoever."

"SOMETIMES MY GUY REALLY DOESN'T WANT TO WEAR A CONDOM. ANY SUGGESTIONS?"

Try the Reality Female Condom, which is made of polyurethane, a highly durable material and a great alternative to latex.

What our customers say:

"They look so big and strange at first, but only because you are comparing them with men's condoms. But they have totally changed my sex life. Since I use condoms as my birth control, in the back of my mind I'm always nervous about trusting the man to be in charge of the condom while having sex. But the Reality condom helps me let go and enjoy sex without any worry."

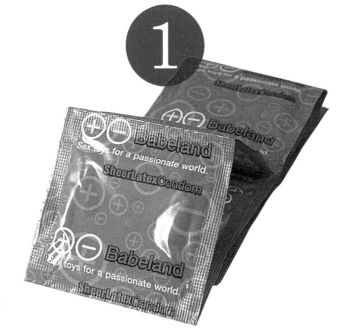

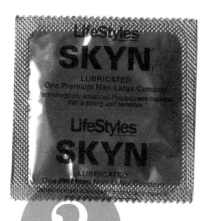

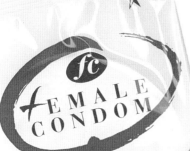

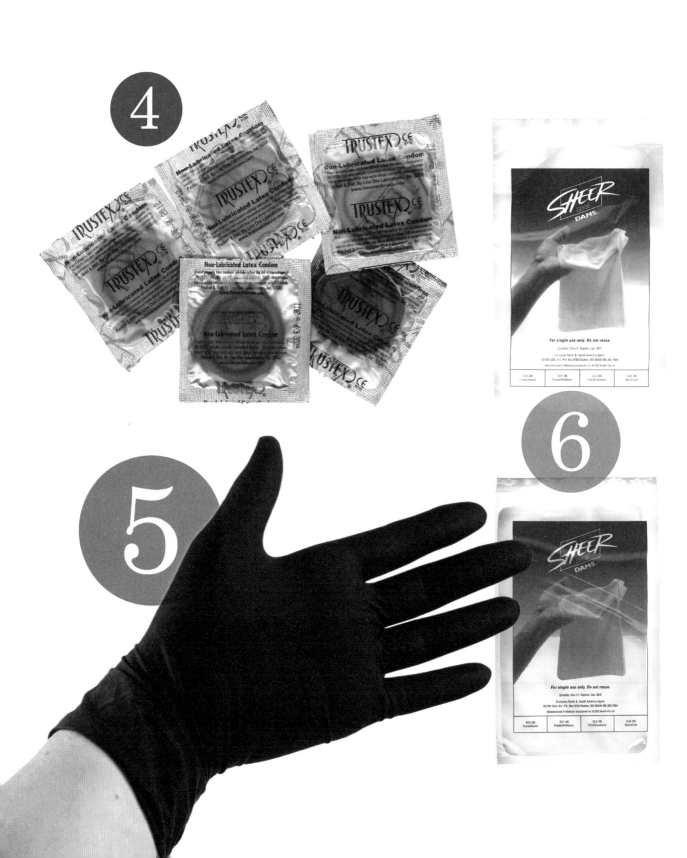

④ "I WANT FULL COLOR!"

Try colored Trustex condoms; these are the best nonlubricated condoms we've seen. Neither lubed nor powdered, they have no taste and are some of the strongest out there. Super for blow jobs or any occasion where you want to provide your own lubrication.

What our customers say:

"These condoms, hands down, are the best condoms for toys. They make for easy cleanup with your vibes and dils, but best of all there is no lube residue on the toys after you peel the condom off!"

⑤ "WHAT'S A GOOD GLOVE FOR FISTING?"

Snap on sexy Black Dragon latex gloves for the business of pleasure. Use these gloves as a barrier for safe sex, keep your hands smooth for penetration, or to indulge your latex fetish to your heart's content. Deliciously smooth all over.

What our customers say:

"I couldn't believe these were latex when I tried them on. They are powder-free, which is a plus. They are so silky and smooth and non-sticky that they are far superior to regular latex gloves. And black is so much sexier than your standard off-white medical latex gloves. I know it sounds ridiculous, but since I bought these, I find myself practicing safe sex far more often than before because I look forward to putting them on."

⑥ "WHAT ABOUT DENTAL DAMS? WHAT'S GOOD?"

Thinner and larger than traditional dental dams, Glyde's silky ultrathin latex lets you experience more and worry less during cunnilingus and analingus. Dimensions are 6" x 10". Available in cream (vanilla-flavored) or black (cola-flavored).

What our customers say:

"I love it! The Glyde dam has added a whole new dimension to our fun. My husband loves the silky texture, and I love making him happy performing analingus, which I really was never so wild about before."

ASK THE BABES

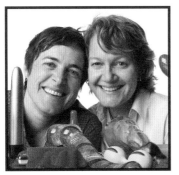

Of course there are speed bumps and potholes all along the highway of your sex life. Instead of calling AAA, we say take a deep breath, slow down your vehicle, and consider a new course. Or maybe even stay the same course but switch to a different gear. We've been addressing common concerns and worries throughout this book, but here are some more questions about sex that we've heard at Babeland over the years. Happy travels!

VIRGINITY ... ?

"I'm a lesbian who's never had sex with a guy. I've done lots of stuff with girls, but my straight friend says I'm still a virgin. Am I?"

— Virgin or Very Experienced

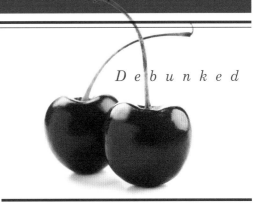

Debunked

IS THE DEFINITION of virginity an intact hymen? If so, a buddy of ours lost her virginity while riding horseback. A simplistic definition of virginity might be exclusively penis/vagina penetration. A more real world definition of virginity is the state of not having experienced sex with another person. If you've had sex that makes your eyes roll and your toes curl and left you collapsed in a heap of tearful release, you're no virgin, no matter who your partner was or what orifice or appendage was involved. It's not just heterosexual intercourse. What is your idea of going all the way? Of physical intimacy? If you're a lifelong sexually active lesbian, you're not a virgin. And don't forget you can cross that line in more than one fashion. Maybe you're a hetero girl who's been having vaginal sex since age twenty, then received your first anal at twenty-seven, then went down on another lady at thirty-two. You "lost your virginity" three times!

"I'm a twenty-six-year-old woman and still a virgin. Am I a freak?"

— V-Card Holder in Boulder

IT MAY BE TRUE that by twenty-six most Americans have made the beast with two backs. But "freak"? We think not. It's a fact that people who lose their virginity later are far more likely to have a good experience. For one thing, we bet that you've been masturbating and know how to get yourself off. This'll help you have more fun with a partner. Perhaps you've had opportunities to do the deed but said no because it wasn't the right time or the right person—mazel tov! You should feel proud about that. But honestly, we think our culture makes way too big a deal about the First Time. It's no wonder that many people wait, what with all the pressure. Try to imagine, though, a situation in which you think sex could be really nice—a friend you've been viewing in a new light? An ex you didn't want to open up to before but now you'd like to try? What changes can you make to bring this vision to life? (See p. 187 for the "Should we do it?" checklist.) And beware of planning One Big Night When You Two Must Have Sex. That kind of pressure can wither the hardest hard-on and tense up any vagina. Instead, try to explore with an open mind and stop if you want—you might do it and you might not. The iffyness can be exciting!

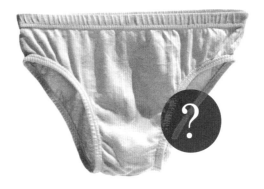

"I'm a seventeen-year-old straight girl. Will my first time having sex hurt? Will I bleed?"

— Worried Wilma

IT MIGHT HURT, but it doesn't have to. Pain during first-time sex is most commonly from two sources: 1) a breaking hymen and/or 2) tense vaginal muscles. You might not have much hymen to start with, but if your hymen does tear during sex, it can hurt at first and bleed a little. But often a woman attributes first-sex pain to the hymen when muscle tension is the culprit. The very best thing you can do your first time is make sure you get warmed up and turned on, and use lots of water-based lube. Being really turned on can diminish pain, so waiting until you're all revved up will help make your first time more enjoyable. Still, it's worth checking: How do fingers feel inside you? Do two fingers in your vagina feel pleasant or painful? If something hurts, back off. The first time is not something to endure through gritted teeth. Take your sweet time.

"I am an eighteen-year-old male. I love my girlfriend, but lately I've only been able to last about one or two minutes before I ejaculate. After that, I go soft and can't get hard again. I feel horrible because I can't please her."

— *Quickie Dickie*

FIRST, TRY TO LET GO of the idea of a right or wrong amount of time. Sex doesn't have to start and end with your erection. A lot of guys your age get hard and ejaculate really fast—that's part of being young and turned on! Second, there are many delightful ways to draw out the fun and satisfy your girlfriend. Maybe you can give her an hour of heavenly oral or a thumpity-fun ride with a vibrator, or let your fingers do the fucking. Or a combo platter of the above. Then finish off the session with your two-minute tango. But if you're truly frustrated and want to make your erection last longer, you can try a cock ring around the cock and balls. The penis gets hard when blood flows into the tissue. Cock rings can extend the duration of your hard-on by slowing the blood flow back out of your penis. Or you can try one of our favorite exercises: When you masturbate, or when you're with a partner, bring yourself close to orgasm and then back off before you come. Literally stop moving. Maybe you

can't stop the volcano from erupting—that's OK—but then pause earlier next time. Like anything else worthwhile: practice, practice, practice.

"I find that when we're about to do the deed, I'm horny as hell and feel ready to go. But then I'm not wet or dripping with desire below deck. Since I'm in my twenties, I feel like I shouldn't need outside lubrication. Is there something I can do to avoid awkward entrances?"

— *Sahara Down There*

THE SOLUTION IS SIMPLE, and its name is "lube." There's absolutely nothing wrong with using lube in your twenties, or at any age. Adding lube can be a regular part of your foreplay. Keep it nearby, even when things are flowing perfectly—it can only help. Dryness is very common. Birth control pills, antihistamines, drugs, and smoking cigarettes can contribute to dryness. Are any of those in your system? Also, make sure you stay hydrated—water can

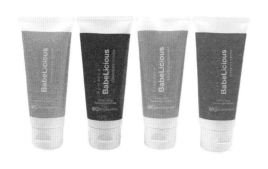

make all the difference. It's also quite possible that you've created a little psych game with yourself: one night you tried to have sex and weren't wet, so the next time you tried to do it you were worried about wetness, and the stress undermined your body's lubrication machinery. Stress about sexual readiness can become a self-fulfilling prophecy, like a guy might have with erections. And people vary a lot in terms of how wet they get.

SEX JUICES BRING UP strong feelings in people, for better or worse. While it would be dreamy if everyone had a big appetite for every juice, sometimes that's not the case. Let him come all over your belly or breasts, so then he's only licking *your* juices later. Or invoking a she-comes-first policy may be the ticket. You get off, then he can pass out after he comes, if he so desires.

SEXUAL IDENTITY...?

"How do I know if I'm gay?"

— *Inquirer in Idaho*

IN OUR CULTURE, we define sexuality by what we do ("I fuck guys") and by what we feel ("but I fantasize about that vampire girl in the *Twilight* movie"). And maybe you're all over the map for the moment— either in your head or in your actions. Be aware of who you find appealing at a party, who you daydream about, who you fall for in the movies, who you picture when you masturbate, and what you picture your-

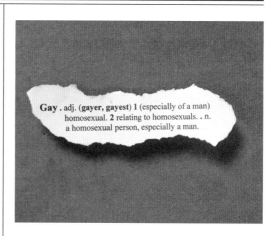

self doing. The ultimate path to a satisfying sex life is knowing what gets your panties wet, literally or metaphorically, and that's a truth you get to discover over a lifetime of changes. You don't have to take on an identity that doesn't feel right to you. In fact, you don't have to take on an identity at all if you don't want to. If you want to have sex with women but don't want to label yourself a lesbian, or bi, or queer, go ahead. *You* get to define who you are—nobody else does. For a lot of us same-sex-loving folk, queer communities are a bonus to the hot sex, but they're not for everyone. What communities do you feel drawn to? There's puh-lenty of support and lots of role models out there. We hope you'll reach a place where your actions and your daydreams are in sync and not at odds.

"My boyfriend's porn habit irks me."

— Looky Here

WHY? Is he more into his porn than you? Whether he's into Guitar Hero or cougar porn, you may feel neglected because it's taking time away from you. If so, talk to him about making sure he's paying attention to the lovely person who's actually in his bed.

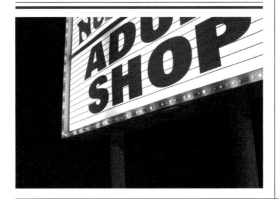

But if you haven't given porn a chance, this can be a classic "if you can't beat 'em, join 'em" situation. We say try to get into it with him on occasion (rent some movies or buy some magazines that turn you on too). Or just chill and let him do his thing. Don't try to change him. If you really can't live with it, well, it might be time to move on to a new partner.

"I'm a woman, and my very butch girlfriend doesn't seem to like to receive. I want to give her pleasure! How can I remedy this? And why is she reluctant?"

— No Diving Allowed

BLESS YOU for wanting to give as well as take. There are a few likely explanations for your sweetie's behavior. Maybe she simply gets off from getting you off. If you look at it that way, then you *are* giving her pleasure. So why is she reluctant? Maybe she's not at ease with the power shift that happens when you're giving and she's receiving. The person getting licked, finger-fucked, or otherwise penetrated is literally in a more vulnerable position. Enjoyment of those acts requires trust and a kind of submission, which just isn't for everyone. Another thought: you say she's very butch, so maybe her relationship with her body and genitals is different from the one you have with yours. Maybe she doesn't want a lot of outside attention on her body, which is understandable, especially if she feels ambivalent about her female parts. You can help by being patient and supportive. Assure her that you find her smokin' hot from head to hangnails and you just want her to feel the sizzle that she's been giving you. Then be open to what she tells you. She might just not want to be on the receiving end of your attentions, and you may have to come to peace with that aspect of your relationship. Or she might let you do more over time. Communication, as always, is key.

"I was really into girls for a while, but now I'm back into guys. What does that make me?"

— *Bi the Way*

SEXUALITY IS FLUID for a lot of people. Some are 100 percent attracted to the same sex or 100 percent attracted to the other sex, but a lot of people feel the sexual buzz in a less compartmentalized way. Labels like gay, straight, and even bisexual can get in the way of your experiencing all the different kinds of lust you have. Labels don't always tell the whole story. Go ahead and love who you love.

"I am worried about my fantasy life. If I fantasize about being forced to have sex, does it mean I'm sick or have really bad self-esteem?"

— *Fantasy Fretter*

FANTASIES ARE NOT REALITY, so don't waste precious life energy worrying about them. Keep in mind that reality is a lot more intense than fantasy, so while in a fantasy you might get off to the idea of being totally overpowered or really hurting someone, in real life some negotiated power exchange would be much healthier. Whatever the fantasy, take the essence of it and use it to spice up what you do in the real world, or just keep it as your own mental playground. In the rare case that your fantasies are truly making you feel that you are at risk for hurting someone (or yourself), then switch gears and find a new train of thought, or seek counseling.

MEDICAL MATTERS ...

"Sometimes sex hurts. Not in an I'm-too-dry-way, but, like, pain."

— *Ouchie in Oregon*

DEFINITELY SEE YOUR DOCTOR, because pain is usually your body's way of asking for attention. Try to notice when it happens (upon first entry of penis/finger/object? In certain positions? At certain times of the month? Does a tampon hurt?) and how it feels (sharp and in one place? Dull and in the entire area?). The more specific you can be, the more a doctor can help you. There are lots of possible—and treatable—causes. You could have a viral or bacterial infection, an internal herpes sore, or tags of hymen tissue that are getting caught and pulled (yee-ouch!). Blocked ducts can get infected or develop cysts. If you've given birth, there might be a tear or sensitive hotspot from the delivery. You should also ask yourself, "Do I want to have sex?" Sometimes after a bad sexual experience (or in anticipation of a bad experience, or with strong feelings of shame), the PC muscles spasm and keep the vagina from opening up—sort of the way your eyelids automatically close when something gets too close. It's a phenomenon called *vaginismus,* and there are treatments for that too.

"Can I have sex with a tampon in?"

— *Room for Two?*

THERE'S ENOUGH ROOM in a fully aroused vagina for both a tampon and a finger/toy/cock, but it'll feel uncomfortable. The tampon might get pushed against your cervix. Why not do some clit rubbing instead! Neither rain nor snow nor menstruation can get in its merry way. Or remove the tampon, put down a towel, and go ahead and bleed. Your cycle is natural, and your lover may find it sexy.

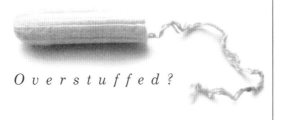

Overstuffed?

"What about douching?"

— *Douche-Curious*

PLEASE AVOID douching and let your body do its own natural cleansing.

"I feel like I get a UTI every time I do it."

— *Sensitive Situation in San Fran*

WOMEN GET urinary tract infections way more often than men do because the female urethra (the tube that leads from pee hole to bladder) is much shorter than the male urethra (which runs the length of his penis). Bacteria gets inside more quickly and easily, making trouble for women. Also, the female pee hole is much closer to the anus than is the male's. (It's anatomical injustice!) Fight this injustice with preventive measures and good hygiene, such as:

• When you go to the bathroom (number one or number two), always **wipe yourself front-to-back** so anal bacteria doesn't get a free ride to your urethra.

• **No backsies-to-frontsies.** In other words, any finger, toy, or penis that's been in your butt is verboten in the pussy due to butt bacteria. An easy solution is to put a condom on anything going in the back door, then remove the condom for a fresh start in the front door.

• **Pee after sex.** You don't have to leap out of bed. Enjoy a postcoital snuggle, but pee within a half hour. This flushes out bacteria.

• **Drink cranberry juice** or take cranberry extract pills. This makes an acidic environment in your bladder, which fights bacterial infection. (Pills are preferable to drinking cranberry juice, which only works if it's totally unsweetened.)

• **Drink lots of water.** Pee flushes you out. Also, don't hold your pee in for too long if you can help it. Make lots of stops on car trips.

If you still have a UTI problem, your doctor can prescribe a low dose of antibiotic that you can take before sex. Remember not to let a UTI go untreated, because it could become a more dangerous kidney infection.

"Can a toy get stuck inside of me?"

— FAO Sports

YOUR VAGINA IS A CLOSED SYSTEM. You can retrieve anything that's up there with a little persistence. Your butt, however, is another story. Nothing should go up your butt that doesn't have a flared base or a string to help you retrieve it. We recommend sticking to objects designed for anal good times. Without a flared base, an object can get pulled in to the point of no return. Hello, emergency room!

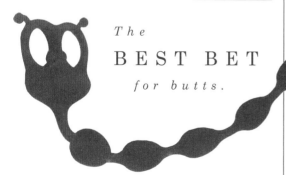

The
BEST BET
for butts.

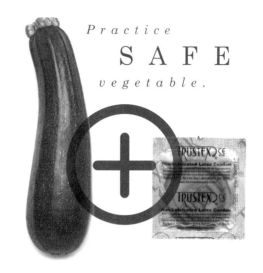

Practice
SAFE
vegetable.

"What's safe to put up my vagina? Can I put a condom on a zucchini?"

— Vegetarian Girl

YES. Vegetables are a fine choice for DIY dildos. Here are some guidelines about what's welcome in the V: nothing too pokey or sharp-edged that could hurt you or tear through the condom (hairbrush, Barbie Doll, spoon). Nothing too fragile that could break (bud vase, lightbulb). Some foods like zucchini or cucumbers have a good shape but yes, they need a condom to keep any dirt out of your pussy.

A tip: gently warm that zucchini in a bowl of water (not a microwave), then put on a condom for warm fun! Speaking of food, putting honey, chocolate sauce, or anything sugary into your V can give you a nasty yeast infection. So avoid this unless you think the yeast infection is really worth the pleasure.

"I seem to have a lower sex drive than my partner, which leaves him frustrated. Should I do it if he wants to and I don't? I love him, but this is causing a strain all around."

— *Sex Drive-ing Me Crazy*

YOU'VE HIT ON a common hotspot. It's definitely tough to find a partner with the exact same level of sex drive—so what to do about the difference? The partner who wants it more may feel undesirable, while the person who wants it less may feel harassed. Definitely talk about it (outside the bedroom) instead of quietly seething. Here are some factors that might be contributing:

Cultural pressure and gender differences.
Keep in mind that our culture trains men to be sexually aggressive. A strong sex drive is considered a sign of masculinity. So men are more likely than women to translate stress, frustration, or anger into sexual desire. Not always, but more likely. For many women, stress is more likely to shut down desire.

Quality over quantity.
It's possible that you feel this imbalance because sex is more satisfying to your partner than to you. Try to work on that with your sweetheart. You can make better sex happen. Keep letting your honey know when it's good (being loud and clear when something is working is a good trick!), and make sure he knows you find him as hot as volcanic lava. This will help him feel more desirable and therefore less rejected.

Timing and old habits.
Maybe your partner always makes a move at bedtime, right before you're falling asleep and when you're exhausted and stressing out over tomorrow's to-do list. Can you consider starting a raunchfest right after work? And, assuming you at least want sex sometimes, why don't you make the first move? It'll go a long way toward making your sweetheart feel like less of a groping, pawing monster.

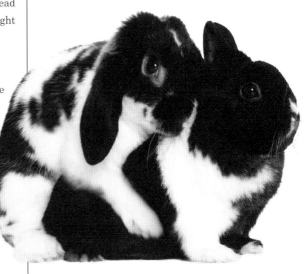

Try it—you might like it.

You shouldn't do anything you don't want to do in bed, full stop. But … if you are feeling so-so, or neutral, or vaguely interested but tired, give him a chance to jump-start your engine. How about a no-strings-attached backrub or pussy licking? Maybe you'll find that your engine gets into gear and you give your partner a green light. If not, then …

Let your partner come for you.

This is an awesome way to balance the sexy scales. If one party wants more partying, let them masturbate. There can still be kissing, or it can be more of a live solo performance for an audience of one, which can be thrilling. It's still a shared and intimate experience, and everybody wins.

"Sometimes I don't even feel like masturbating for weeks (or months) at a time. Is that fucked up?"

— *Meh about Masturbation*

NO. It's not a problem if you don't feel like it's a problem. The last thing you need is peer pressure from yourself. Instead, give yourself permission to take a break for a while. Maybe you'll direct all your sexual energy into the greatest screenplay, sculpture, yearly report, or ten-layer lasagna you've ever made. Are you having partner sex? That might be enough for the time being. Fine. When you're bored or horny enough, maybe you'll want to shake up your wanking life with a new sex toy or position. There's also the possibility that you're just not a very sexual person— there is such a thing as asexual. It's worth noting that there is a continuum of libido, from high to none,

and if it feels good to you, there is no wrong amount. Note, however, that in some cases, having no sex drive for a long stretch can be a red flag for depression. Check in with yourself about that.

"How much sex is normal? How many times a week should we be doing it?"

— *Nervous About Normalcy*

AS OFTEN AS YOU WANT, as long as you're not messing up your life or engaging in risky behavior just to get some. There really is no "normal." What's important is that you're satisfied. Try not to worry about what your friends are doing or how frequently they're doing it. But if you're asking because you're in a steady relationship and feel like you aren't getting enough sex, it's time to stop and assess. What's the main roadblock—stress, time management, a partner who doesn't want to? (See above answer.)

"I hate this woman. I'm not into her looks, her personality, her whole M.O. But Jesus, I'm so hot for her. WTF?"

— *Attracted in Arkansas*

WELCOME TO THE START of many a good sitcom. We hope you see the humor in your own situation. It's called chemistry, and you've got it bad. Physical chemistry doesn't depend on the two of you having the same taste in music or political candidates. Don't spin out in your head about it. Instead, enjoy! If you're really not into this woman, you can let her live in your fantasies. But maybe, just maybe, it's worth exploring this chemistry on a date or two as you expand your idea of who's appealing to you (always a good exercise). Or maybe you two just need to go for it in the copy room after work. Can you get paid overtime for that?

"My live-in boyfriend and I haven't gone at it in six months. What do we do?"

— Dry Spell in Kalispell

SOMETIMES SHARING a bed can feel like a very lonely experience, but it's up to you to bust out of a slump. Have you talked about your situation? (Preferably outside the bedroom, over coffee in the

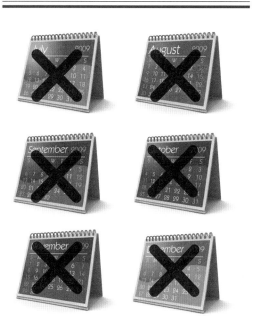

kitchen, maybe.) Do you know why this is happening? Stress? No time alone? Bad feelings? Laziness? The best thing you can do—and it can be really fun—is to start over from square one. Court each other. Go on a date where you're only allowed to make out. Take things really slow and trust that the spark will come back. Maybe go over our "Yes/No/Maybe" list (p. 114) and pick one activity for that night. And remember, intimacy and foreplay start before you get to the bedroom. Do you kiss your boyfriend on the back of the neck while he's dicing potatoes for your dinner? If not, try it. Do you take responsibility for revving up your own sexual energy and bringing it to him, say, by talking dirty or coming on to him? Maybe you'll end up unleashing the sexual connection you two shared before he moved in.

"Two weeks out of the month, I'm rubbing against corners of tables. The other two weeks, I'm like, 'Get away from me!'"

— Unbalanced Urges

ONE WORD: hormones. These powerful chemicals rule us more than we'd care to admit. The two weeks in which you're secretly violating your furniture are probably early- to mid-cycle, around ovulation time. You're at your most fertile, and Mother Nature is trying to get you knocked up. Start keeping track of the horny vs. "hell no!" days on your calendar. Enjoy your lively libido when it kicks in. Be patient with yourself on the off days. Warn your partner about this fluctuation so they don't take it personally when you're not into it and can build anticipation for when you are.

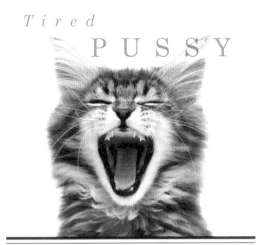

Tired PUSSY

"I'm so bored with my long-term partner."

— Malaised Mojo in Minnesota

OUR FIRST QUESTION IS "Why?" Do you feel more like best friends? That can be a desire-killer. Sometimes it's hard to want what you already have. And if you think you know everything about your partner, where's the mystery? Mystery, uncertainty, and newness are all good for desire. You might feel like you threw those qualities out the window when you chose stability. But you didn't, and you can cultivate their regrowth. Couples come into our shops all the time looking to add some freshness and sparkle to their coupling—we love this! A date night spent exploring in a grown-up candy store does a couple good. ("Oh, I didn't know you thought blindfolds were hot." "Hey, would you ever strap this dildo on?") Suddenly you're seeing your beloved in a new way. That can help. If you're not near an adult toy store, snuggle up online together (www.Babeland.com). The "Yes/No/Maybe" list (p. 114) can help. See also the Mojo Jump-Starter at right.

MOJO JUMP-STARTER

Instead of asking yourself why your long-term partner seems about as sexy as a long wait at the airport baggage claim, turn your gaze within. Ask yourself, "When do I feel sexy? When do I turn myself on?" Put pen to paper and make a list. Maybe the answers are:

- When I play the guitar
- **When I dress up in my red Prada pumps**
- When I talk to my college friends and we dish
- **When I'm learning a new skill**
- When I walk down the street like I own it
- **When I work on something creative**

OK. Now ask yourself when you last played the guitar, wore your red pumps, called your friends, took a class, walked tall, etc.? If you can turn yourself back on, you'll be one step closer to working your mojo on your favorite lovah–or someone you haven't even met yet.

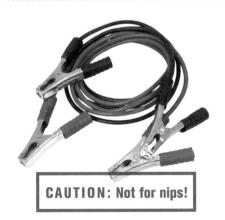

CAUTION: Not for nips!

GETTING ANAL...

"My boyfriend of many years is more into anal sex than I am. I've tried, but it makes me feel like I'm going to the bathroom."

— *Exit Only*

IF BY ANAL SEX you mean a penis up the butt, it's probably too much too soon. Start with a rim job, a finger, a butt plug, or some beads. Go slowly, breathing to relax and see if you don't find that it feels kinda good. Keep exploring that feeling. And who knows? Maybe at some point you'll want to invite your boyfriend back in.

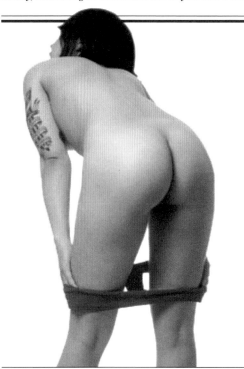

"Recently, I was out with a female business client. We had some drinks, then a great conversation about anal sex and toys. I came home on fire and my guy spanked and licked my ass until I came. Why did I get so aroused from talking about anal play with a woman?"

— *A-Hole New World?*

CAMARADERIE IS freeing. It feels great to open up to another person about something taboo, and to be heard and understood. The math equation: anal sex + girl-on-girl dirty talk + business client you can't date + alcohol = a lot of taboo and naughtiness for one night. It was exciting! And it took you out of your comfort zone! It got you hot! This is a great example of bringing the energy and zing from the outside world into the bedroom with your longtime partner. If it works, work it.

"I really like anal play. My boyfriend started off using his fingers, then I got into butt plugs, and now we have anal sex regularly. Will I be in adult diapers by the time I hit fifty?"

— Butt Seriously

YOUR SPHINCTER MUSCLES are getting more elastic and relaxed, and that's a good thing. If anything, you're toning them—not stretching them. As long as you're not forcing anything in there, you're not doing any damage.

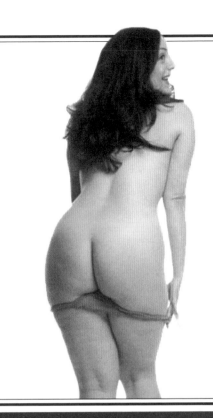

FERTILITY, PREGNANCY ...

"Ever since we started trying for a kid, I can't tell you how disinterested I am in sex."

— Trying Times

THIS IS A COMMON complaint. Goal-oriented sex is not terribly erotic. If you've been trying for a while, stress, shame, and blame can start creeping—or pouring—into your bedroom. ("What if I'm broken inside?" "What if I'm doing this wrong?" "What if I never get to be a parent?" "Why can't he deliver the swimmers I need?") Not very sexy or relaxing, yet you want to work together to keep trying. A few helpful tips:

• Make sure you still **enjoy sex play** like cunnilingus, kissing, or kink. Don't get so focused on intercourse that you forget to keep it hot.

• **Enjoy the days of the month that you are not trying** for a baby. Those are days when sex is just for fun—if you take breaks from sex during those times, sex will start to feel too single-minded.

• **Take turns making sex requests** that bring the fun back. ("Tuesday you tie me up, Thursday I tie you up").

• Unless you're in a big hurry, **enjoy a full year of trying**. If you're still not pregnant, see a fertility doctor to make sure everything's in working order. If it's not, you can make a game plan. A doc visit can remove some of the stress and pressure and make you feel like you have an ally.

"Can I get pregnant from sex during my period?"

— Red Tide Rising

YES—it's unlikely, but possible. Some women have mid-month bleeding that they think is their Aunt Flo, but it isn't. So those are not pregnancy-proof days to have sex. If you have unprotected sex at the end of your period, and then you ovulate early, the sperm can hang out until the egg arrives on the scene. Those little tadpoles can live for five days up in your puss. So don't get arrogant and swear, "Oh, I know my cycle." You could be wrong, or you can have a wacky cycle at any time. That's almost as bad as a guy saying "I promise I'll pull out."

"Sex during pregnancy— is it OK? Is a dick knocking on my cervix harmful?"

— Knocked Up and Needing It

CHECK WITH your doctor to make sure yours is not a high-risk pregnancy. But bun-in-oven sex is generally safe and great—that is, if you want to have it. Hormones, nausea, aches, and exhaustion cause some women to put sex on a shelf for a while, especially in the first three months. (Don't worry, horniness returns!) Upped estrogen and increased sensitivity turn others into prenatal tigresses. Breasts get a lot bigger (fun!) and you can't get more pregnant. A dick near the cervix is fine, unless it's hurting you. As you get bigger, rear-entry positions with you two on your sides can feel good (see positions on p. 199). Oral and manual sex are good ideas too (in general, but particularly right now). Toward the end, some couples use sex to help induce labor. Just don't have sex after your water breaks, as that could cause infection.

"I just had a kid, and I'm finding sex painful. How do I get back into the swing of things?"

— Feeling Rusty

AFTER GIVING BIRTH, your doctor will tell you not to have sex for up to six weeks. Even after the waiting period, a lot of new moms still experience pain when being penetrated. You may be tensing up out of fear of being hurt—you just pushed a whole baby out, and your vagina may not be as ready as your libido to resume having sex. In this case you and your partner need to take it easy and let your recovery (physical and emotional) take its course. If you tore or had an episiotomy, the pain could be coming from that injury, and that can take quite a while to completely heal. Masturbation is a great way to get reacquainted with your parts as they return to normal, and Kegel exercises (see p. 23) will help you regain internal muscle

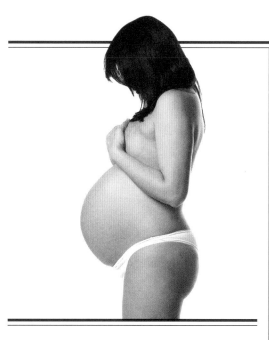

"I'm having a lot of trouble finding myself sexy since giving birth."

— Nobody's MILF

WE ARE CONSTANTLY bombarded by images of beauty—it can be a challenge to feel good about how you look even when you're fresh and twenty-three! And we have high expectations for a libido that's always revved up and ready. After your body has been through something transformative like pregnancy and childbirth, it's a good time to give yourself a break. You don't have to be a sex machine. Get some sleep, get back in touch with what turns you on, and your erotic energy will start to matter more to you than whatever physical imperfections you see. You're a mom, and you are sexy in a new, powerful way. And a big P.S.: Childbirth can actually make sex better! A lot of women say they have bigger, more full-body orgasms after vaginal birth.

tone. When you're ready to explore penetration, start with (clean) fingers. Use lots of lube, as hormones can make you dry. Work your way up over time from fingers to dildo or penis. Patience, patience, patience. And if the pain continues, talk to your doctor.

PARENTING ...

"How does anyone have sex after children?"

— No Time for Nooky

UM, QUIETLY? Why do you think they made Saturday morning cartoons? And don't feel guilty if you let the baby cry a little longer while you're finishing your strokes (and we don't mean golf or tennis). Happy parents are better parents. Try to make nooky a priority so you don't end up resenting the kids. It's

not their fault! You're gonna have to get creative. Do it fast and dirty in the laundry room during Junior's nap. Get a babysitter. Send the kids to a neighbor for an hour or two. Rent a hotel room (sexy!). And don't forget how to masturbate either. When kids are at school or asleep, lock the door and sneak in some vibe time. Small children are demanding, but only temporarily. It's easy to forget that they really will get older and you won't be at their beck and call forever. We promise, you will have sex again. It just may have to be a quickie during *Sesame Street*.

OLDER SEX ...

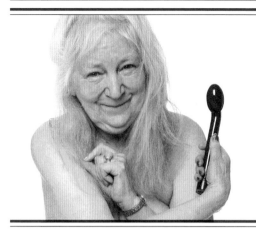

"I just turned 60 and hit menopause. My sex drive plummeted. Is this the end for me?"

— *Silver Foxy*

NO, DEFINITELY NOT. Like pregnancy, menopause is a transitional state when your hormone recipe is changing. Some women get horny, and some women get decidedly unhorny. And even the unhorny ones like yourself tend to find the state temporary and get back into sex later. During menopause, your estrogen level goes down, which reduces your natural vaginal juices and genital blood flow. But water-based lube can help increase wetness, and masturbation (if you're up for it) gets your blood pumping. Kegel exercises keeps your sex parts toned. Classic menopause symptoms like headaches, insomnia, and hot flashes can be annoying at best and debilitating at worst, but they're not permanent. Talk to your doctor to see if modern medicine is offering something helpful in the meantime. But no, you don't need to send your pussy to the Smithsonian as a lost relic of the past.

"Can women take Viagra or Cialis?"

— *Feeling Left Out*

THERE ARE REPORTS of recreational use of these drugs by women, but there's no proof that Viagra or Cialis are effective for gals. They can be dangerous if taken without a doctor's guidance. Yes, these meds increase the blood flow, but they won't suddenly give you a ragin' sex drive if that's what you're after. They have a lot of caffeine and can also cause a major headache the next day.

"Is sex still good after seventy? Is seventy the new sixty?"

— *Senior Humper*

YES, SENIOR CITIZENS CAN still get saucy— and they do. What did you think retirement was for—knitting? Actually, the increase in free time often makes for more sensual, unhurried loving than in the working-hard-and-raising-kids days. For many seniors, it takes longer to reach orgasm, but this helps free us from getting too goal-oriented (an approach we think is the best at any age). You might need to do the deed earlier in the day, when you have more energy. And keep some lube on the bedside table next to your reading glasses. Condoms, too. Though pregnancy is no longer an issue, you still need to practice safe sex unless you are monogamous and have both been tested for STIs.

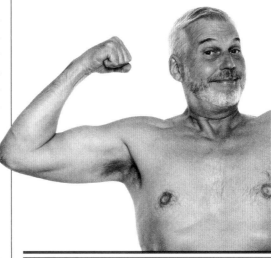

"Can men use Viagra forever?"

— Poppin' in Poughkeepsie

IF THE DOCTOR SAYS so, yes. Go for it. But remember, Viagra only helps the sexual mechanics through increased blood flow. It does not treat libido, which might be winding down as a gent approaches "forever." Even a soft penis is sensitive and fun to play with. And don't forget that sex at any age does not have to mean cock-in-pussy. The later years are a great time to explore nongenital touch. If you're getting thrills and the feeling of intimacy from your body—with foot rubs, romantic bubble baths—who needs Viagra?

AND FINALLY ...

"Can sex keep getting better throughout the rest of my life?"

— Lifetime Groover

YES. ALWAYS, YES. Look at it this way: you started talking at a young age, but your conversations were basic and just got the job done. As you got older, your experience and vocabulary increased, and you became a better conversationalist. (You're probably a better listener too.) Sex is like a conversation. It's a form of interplay and communication that's surprising and satisfying (or deep or quick or comforting or funny). And the better you know yourself, the better you'll be able to express your desires with another person. Sometimes we want theatrical, kinky, complicated sexual encounters. And sometimes we want kissy, lovey, heart-connection lovemaking. So as long as you're honest with yourself and keep your ears open to your partner and the world around you, your skills and good times should keep on keeping on.

RESOURCES

You can always come to babeland.com for information and answers to questions (updated regularly), but here are some additional resources for specific questions and interests.

BDSM

The Eulenspiegel Society
tes.org
The oldest and largest BDSM education and support group in New York City.

FetLife
fetlife.com
A free social network for the kinky (bondage, BDSM, and fetish) community. Similar to Facebook and MySpace but run by kinksters.

Lesbian Sex Mafia
lesbiansexmafia.org
Founded in 1981, the Lesbian Sex Mafia is one of the oldest women's BDSM support and education groups in the country.

The Society of Janus
soj.org
San Francisco–based support and education organization for people interested in learning about BDSM. SOJ provides an opportunity to meet others with similar interests in a safe, relaxed atmosphere.

The Submit Party
submitparty.com
Premier BDSM and sex party for women and trans folks, located in New York City.

BODY IMAGE

Bellies Are Beautiful Body-Positive Gallery
belliesarebeautiful.com
Private project by Stacy Bias dedicated to positive body image for all people. Bellies Are Beautiful is a celebrative, but not exploitative, collection of user-submitted bellies of all sizes, shapes, colors, and genders.

Big Fat Deal
bfdblog.com
A body-positivity blog that welcomes people who are trying to lose weight as well as people who are happy to be whatever weight they happen to be.

Health at Every Size
haescommunity.org
Movement based on the simple premise that the best way to improve health is to honor your body. It supports people in adopting health habits for the sake of health and well-being (rather than weight control).

Kate Harding's Shapely Prose
kateharding.net
Kate Harding is a Chicago-based writer, editor, and contributor to Fatshionista, Shakesville, and Salon's Broadsheet.

DATING

Curve Personals
curvepersonals.com
Lesbian personals from the nation's best-selling lesbian magazine.

Lavalife

lavalife.com

Free dating, personals, love, romance, and more.

Nerve Personals

personals.nerve.com

Free personals from Nerve.

Ok Cupid

okcupid.com

Free dating service with hundreds of thousands of online users.

Plenty of Fish

plentyoffish.com

Free online dating and match-making service for singles. Daily active members number 900,000.

DISABILITY

Deaf Queer Resource Center

deafqueer.org

Resources and information for, by, and about the deaf lesbian, gay, bisexual, and transgender communities.

National Sexuality Resource Center

nsrc.sfsu.edu /

Creates content, leads training sessions, and guides the development of a new sexuality movement, founded on the unique concept of sexual literacy—a positive, integrated, and holistic view of sexuality from a social justice perspective.

The Sexual Health Network

sexualhealth.com

Dedicated to providing easy access to sexuality information, education, support, and other resources.

FEMINISM

Bitch Magazine

bitchmagazine.org

Provides commentary on our media-driven world from a feminist perspective.

Feministing

feministing.com

Feministing provides a platform for women to comment, analyze, influence, and connect on issues that affect their lives and futures.

Feminists for Free Expression

ffeusa.org

A group of diverse feminists working to preserve the individual's right and responsibility to read, listen, view, and produce materials of her choice.

HEALTH AND SAFETY

Kink-Aware Professionals via the National Coalition for Sexual Freedom

www.ncsfreedom.org

A privately funded, non-profit service dedicated to providing the kink community with referrals to psychotherapeutic, medical, and legal professionals who are knowledgeable about and sensitive to diverse expressions of sexuality.

The National Domestic Violence Hotline

ndvh.org, 800-799-SAFE (7233), 800-787-3224 (TTY)

Established in 1996 as a component of the Violence Against Women Act (VAWA) passed by Congress. The Hotline answers a variety of calls and is a resource for domestic violence advocates, government officials, law enforcement agencies, and the general public.

Planned Parenthood

plannedparenthood.org

Information and resources covering sexual and reproductive health topics. Research on sexual health problems and directory of health centers in the U.S.

The Sexual Health Network

www.sexualhealth.com

Dedicated to providing easy access to sexuality information, education, support, and other resources.

INTERSEX

Intersex Society of North America

isna.org

Includes contact information, medical information, articles, newsletter, bibliography, store, FAQs, and writings about the intersex condition.

LESBIAN/GAY ORGANIZATIONS

Gay & Lesbian Alliance Against Defamation (GLAAD)

glaad.org

Dedicated to promoting and ensuring fair, accurate, and inclusive representation of people and events in the media as a means of eliminating homophobia and discrimination based on gender identity and sexual orientation.

National Gay and Lesbian Task Force (NGLTF)

thetaskforce.org

Promotes civil rights for gay, lesbian, bisexual, and transgender people. Includes federal and state organizing news, issue backgrounders, and analysis.

National Center for Lesbian Rights (NCLR)

nclrights.org

Legal resource center committed to advancing the rights and safety of lesbians. Litigation, public policy advocacy, free legal advice, and counseling.

PROFESSIONAL ORGANIZATIONS

American Association of Sexuality Educators, Counselors, and Therapists

aasect.org

A not-for-profit, interdisciplinary professional organization. These individuals share an interest in promoting understanding of human sexuality and healthy sexual behavior.

Sexuality Information and Education Council of the United States

siecus.org

Founded in 1964 to provide education and information about sexuality and sexual and reproductive health.

The Society for the Scientific Study of Sexuality

sexscience.org

International organization dedicated to the advancement of knowledge about sexuality. It is the oldest organization of professionals interested in the study of sexuality in the United States.

SAFER SEX

Centers for Disease Control and Prevention

cdc.gov

Online source for credible health information.

Gay Men's Health Crisis

gmhc.org

HIV and AIDS information from the world's oldest HIV/AIDS service organization.

Lesbian Health & Research Center

lesbianhealthinfo.org

University of California center for lesbian health issues, research, information, and events.

The Safer Sex Page

safersex.org

A free information and referral switchboard providing anonymous, accurate, nonjudgmental information about all aspects of sex.

National STD & AIDS Hotlines

800-227-8922 or 800-342-2437

Information and referrals to free and low-cost public clinics. Operators can answer general questions on prevention, symptoms, transmission, and treatment of sexually transmitted diseases. Open 24 hours.

SEX INFORMATION, EDUCATION, AND CLASSES

About.com: Sexuality

sexuality.about.com

General information on sex and sexuality.

The Body Electric School

bodyelectric.org

Offers workshops and classes on Tantra.

Center for Sex & Culture

sexandculture.org

Provides nonjudgmental, sex-positive sexuality education and support to diverse populations by means of classes and workshops.

Our Bodies Ourselves

ourbodiesourselves.org

Our Bodies Ourselves, also known as the Boston Women's Health Book Collective, is a nonprofit women's health education, advocacy, and consulting organization.

San Francisco Sex Information

sfsi.org

Trains people to become sex educators and operates a free information and referral switchboard. Provides free, confidential, accurate, nonjudgmental information about sex and reproductive health.

Society for Human Sexuality

sexuality.org

Provides positive and helpful information on all forms of human sexuality.

Tantric Sex

tantra.com

Features videos, position illustrations, techniques, and personals.

SEXUAL ABUSE

Gender Education & Advocacy

gender.org

A national organization focused
on the needs, issues, and concerns of gender-variant people
in human society.

Generation 5

generationfive.org

Nonprofit organization that
brings together diverse community leaders working to end
child sexual abuse within five
generations.

**National Sexual Violence
Resource Center (NSVRC)**

nsvrc.org

Serves as the nation's principal
information and resource center
regarding all aspects of sexual
violence.

**Rape, Abuse & Incest National
Network (RAINN)**

rainn.org

The nation's largest anti-sexual
assault organization.

**TRANSGENDER/
TRANSSEXUAL/
GENDERQUEER**

**Callen-Lorde Community
Health Center**

callen-lorde.org

New York City's only primary

health care center dedicated
to meeting the health needs of
the lesbian, gay, bisexual, and
transgender communities and
people living with HIV/AIDS—
regardless of any patient's
ability to pay.

Female-to-Male International

ftmi.org

Organization serving the female-
to-male community.

Gender Identity Project

gaycenter.org/gip

Works to foster the healthy development of transgender and gender
nonconforming people, partners,
family, and community.

Gender Talk

gendertalk.com

Largest radio archive of progres-
sive, trans-friendly radio programs.

**Kate Bornstein's Blog
for Teens, Freaks,
and Other Outlaws**

katebornstein.typepad.com

Kate Bornstein is a transgendered
author, playwright, and performance artist.

**Transgender Awareness
Training and Advocacy**

tgtrain.org

Transgender training for health
care providers, medical students,
and human service providers.

Transgender Law Center

transgenderlawcenter.org

Civil rights organization advocat-
ing for transgender communities.

YOUTH

**Coalition for
Positive Sexuality**

positive.org

Works to give teens the information they need to take care
of themselves and in so doing
affirm their decisions about sex,
sexuality, and reproductive
control, and aims to facilitate
dialogue in public schools on
condom availability and sex
education.

Go Ask Alice

goaskalice.columbia.edu/

Question and answers on
many topics, with a health focus.
From Columbia University's
Health Education Program, with
a searchable database.

Scarleteen

scarleteen.com

Sex-positive sex education.
Articles, advice, accurate
information, and interactive
media for young adults.

Sex, Etc.

sexetc.org

Info and advice on sex, love
and relationships, pregnancy,
birth control and condoms,
STDs, and more. Published by
Answer, a part of the Center
for Applied Psychology at
Rutgers University.

INDEX

Page numbers in italics refer to illustrations.

REFERENCES

Our years of experience and fabulous staff helped inform most of this book's content, but the following books also provided invaluable help.

Berman, Laura. *Real Sex for Real Women*. London: Dorling Kindersley, 2008.

Blue, Adrianne. "The Kiss." *The Independent*, June 1, 1996

Cavanah, Claire and Rachel Venning. *Sex Toys 101: A Playfully Uninhibited Guide*. New York: Fireside, 2003.

Chalker, Rebecca. *The Clitoral Truth: The Secret World at Your Fingertips*. New York: Seven Stories Press, 2000.

Cosmopolitan. *Cosmo's Guide to Red-Hot Sex*. New York: Hearst, 2008.

Desalle, Marie and Marcy Michaels. *The Low Down on Going Down: How to Give Her Mind-Blowing Oral Sex*. New York: Broadway, 2004.

Jablonski, Nina G. *Skin: A Natural History*. Berkeley and Los Angeles: University of California Press, 2006.

Joannides, Paul. *Guide to Getting It On*. Oregon: Goofy Foot Press, 2009.

Semans, Anne and Cathy Winks. *The Good Vibrations Guide to Sex*. San Francisco: Cleis Press, 2002

Taylor, Emma and Lorelei Sharkey. *Sex: How to Do Everything*. London: Dorling Kindersley, 2008.

Waxman, Jayme. *Getting Off: A Woman's Guide to Masturbation*. Jackson, Tennessee: Seal Press, 2007

ACKNOWLEDGMENTS

Crafting a sex book is no one-night stand, and for all of their hard work and long nights writing, photographing, designing, and illustrating sex, we'd like to thank our contributors. Thank you to Charlie Melcher and the team at Melcher Media, especially Holly Rothman and Coco Joly, for producing *Moregasm*. Thank you to Jessica Vitkus for her careful research and hilarious writing. Thanks to Sarah Small and her talented crew for shooting such beautiful photos. Thank you to the gifted Paul Kepple of Headcase Design for art directing the book, and to Anders Wenngren for his cool illustrations. Special thanks to the good people at Avery Books for believing in this project, especially Bill Shinker, Lauren Marino, and Brianne Mulligan.

A big thank you to all the Babelanders who helped create this book, availing themselves to help with everything from providing product photography and giving interviews to modeling for us: Kelly Arbor, Jennyrose Churchill-Ernst, Dallas, Darlinda Just Darlinda, Pamela Doan, Mary Hoffer, Kathi Ko, Jennifer May, Aislinn Race, Anne Semans, Brandi Sims, Lacy Warner, Laura Weide, Abby Weintraub, Aimee Wiercinki, and Emily Wright. Thanks to Alex McCabe. Finally, thank you to everyone who appeared in this book. You're all amazing, and thanks to you, the world is a sexier place.

Melcher Media would like to thank David E. Brown, Caroline Brownell, Amelie Cherlin, Cheryl della Pietra, Barbara Gogan, Sam Lambert, Lauren Nathan, Lia Ronnen, Jessi Rymill, Dr. Michael Singer, Lindsey Stanberry, Alex Tart, Shoshana Thaler, Rebecca Weiner, and Megan Worman.

PHOTOGRAPHY CREDITS

All photographs © Sarah Small except as noted: p.22: Steve Goodwin; p.37 (left to right): Gord Horne, Thomas Milewski, Susan Trigg; p.39 (clockwise from top left): courtesy of iStock, Danny Smythe, Emrah Turudu, Donald Erickson, Sarah Small, courtesy of iStock, Dan Nichols, courtesy of iStock, Cindy England; p.54: Nicolas Loran; p.65: Anastasiya Maksymenko; p.67 (middle image): courtesy of iStock; p.91: Nicholas Monu; p.94 (left to right): David Russell, courtesy of iStock p.96: Mike Tolstoy; p.107: Doug Cannell; p. 115 (clockwise from top left): Sharon Dominick, Mark Evans, Todd Taulman, Fabio Cecconello, courtesy of iStock, John Hoist, Daniel Heywood, courtesy of Babeland, Sarah Small, Mark Aplet, Camilla Wisbaver, Viorika Prikhodko, Andrzej Tokarski, Emre Ogan; p.124: Martin Carlsson; p.125: Andrew Johnson; p.126 (left to right): Kenny Haner, courtesy of iStock; p.127 (left to right): Johanna Goodyear, Simon Askham; p.130: Olga Ekaterincheva; p.132: Marc Dietrich; p.133: Rich Legg; p.135: Tomasz Darul; p.140-141 (left to right): Jill Fromer, Barbra Bergfeldt; p.144: Momoko Takeda; p.147: Daniel Heywood; p.152: Ken Cameron (middle image), Daniela Jovanovska-Hristovska (hands); p.155: courtesy of iStock; p.157: courtesy of iStock; p.160: Libby Chapman; p.161: courtesy of iStock; p.167: courtesy of iStock; p.177: courtesy of iStock; p.173: Alexey Stiop; p.184–185: Anandha Krishnan; p.230-231: Tomaz Levstek; p.234 (top to bottom): Christoph Achenbach, Ariusz Nawrocki, courtesy of Babeland; p.235 (top to bottom): Leve Dolgatshjov, Kevin Sharpe, Nick Schlax; p.238 (left image): Nieves Mares Pagan; p.239 (left to right): Jenny Swanson, Paul Rosado; p.246: Jacob Wackerhausen; p.247: Clayton Hansen; p.249 (left to right): courtesy of Babeland, Mark Wragg; p.250: Bonnie Schupp; p.252: courtesy of iStock; p.253 (left to right): courtesy of Babeland, courtesy of iStock, courtesy of Babeland; p.254: Jan Emil Christiansen; p.256-257 (left to right): Lev Mel, Butinova Elena, Jolanta Dabrowska; p.261: Maksim Toome; p.263: Frank Camhi. Product photography throughout is courtesy of Babeland.

Persons whose photos appear in this book are over the age of eighteen.

ABOUT THE CONTRIBUTORS

Jessica Vitkus (writer) worked for many years as a journalist at MTV news—where she wrote the infamous "Boxers or briefs?" question for the town meeting with President Clinton. Since then she has shown her sexy side by writing an advice book for young people called *Smart Sex*. She's expressed her crafty side writing for Martha Stewart magazines and authoring a book of projects called *AlternaCrafts*. And she's let loose her funny side producing and writing for *Pop-Up Video*, *The Daily Show with Jon Stewart*, Public Radio International, CNN, Sundance Channel, and more. Jessica is currently producing for MTV's hit series *16 and Pregnant*.

Sarah Small (photographer) was trained at the Rhode Island School of Design and resides in Brooklyn, New York. She has taught darkroom photography to both high-school students and adults and currently teaches Portrait Photography at the Parsons School of Design. Her work has appeared in publications including *Vogue*, *Life*, and *The New York Times*. Her images have been exhibited in the U.S. and internationally at venues including The Corcoran Gallery, Caprice Horn Gallery, and The Australian Center for Photography. She has been the recipient of numerous awards, and was recently named by *American Photo* as one of the "Top 13 Emerging Photographers" working today.

Paul Kepple and *Scotty Reifsnyder* (designer) are better known as *Headcase Design*, an award-winning graphic design and illustration studio based in Philadelphia. Their work has been recognized by such publications as the *AIGA'S 365* and *50 Books/50 Covers*, *American Illustration*, *Communication Arts*, and *Print*.

This book was produced by:
Melcher Media
124 West 13th Street
New York, NY 10011
www.melcher.com

Publisher: Charles Melcher
Associate Publisher: Bonnie Eldon
Editor in Chief: Duncan Bock
Senior Editor and Project Manager: Holly Rothman
Editorial Assistant: Coco Joly
Production Director: Kurt Andrews
Production Associate: Daniel del Valle